Embarrass Less

EMBARRASS LESS

A PRACTICAL GUIDE FOR DOCTORS, NURSES, STUDENTS AND HOSPITALS

Michael W. Perry

INKLING BOOKS   AUBURN   2016

DESCRIPTION

Although hospitalized patients rarely say so, embarrassment is one of their greatest fears. This book examines their concerns and explains how caregivers can reduce those fears, often to the vanishing point. Patients will become more comfortable and cooperative. Care will go more smoothly and efficiently,

DEDICATION

To all the patients who, when I knew so little, were kind enough to be patient.

LIBRARY CATALOGING DATA

Title: *Embarrass Less: A Practical Guide for Doctors, Nurses, Students and Hospitals*
Author: Michael W. Perry (1948–).

DESCRIPTION:

164 pages with 25 pictures. Photos from Adobe Stock, Big Stock Photos, Deposit Photos, Pixabay, and Yoninah on Wikimedia. Others from individual sources.
Size: 6 x 9 x 0.35 inches, 229 x 152 x 9 mm. Weight: 0.5 pounds, 230 grams.
Library of Congress Control Number: 2016915513
With the exception of Beth, who was my cousin, and Binky, his actual nickname, to ensure privacy all the names in this book are not actual names.

BISAC SUBJECT HEADINGS

MED011000 Medical / Caregiving
MED024000 Medical / Education & Training
MED058050 Medical / Nursing / Fundamentals & Skills
MED058140 Medical / Nursing / Nurse & Patient

ISBN ASSIGNMENTS

Trade paperback: 978-1-58742-092-4
Epub reflowable: 978-1-58742-093-1 (iBookstore)
Epub fixed-layout: 978-1-58742-094-8 (iBookstore)
Kindle reflowable: 978-1-58742-095-5 (Amazon)
Kindle fixed layout: 978-1-58742-096-2 (Amazon)
Other: 978-1-58742-097-9 (additional digital editions)

PUBLISHER INFORMATION

Print edition printed on acid-free paper in the U.S.A. and other countries.
Body text is Adobe Caslon Pro. Chapter headings are Minion Pro.
First edition. First printing, October 2016
Publisher: Inkling Books, Auburn, AL 36830
Internet: http://www.InklingBooks.com/

CONTENTS

MY NIGHTS WITH LEUKEMIA

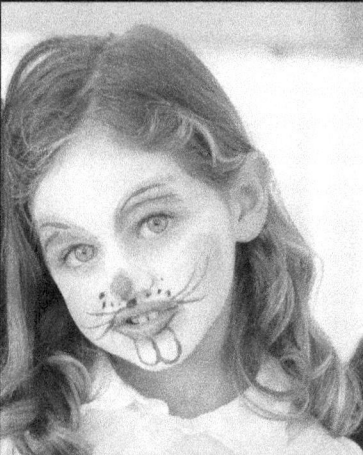

CARING FOR CHILDREN WITH CANCER
MICHAEL W. PERRY

Curing What Ails Hospital
Nursing Morale

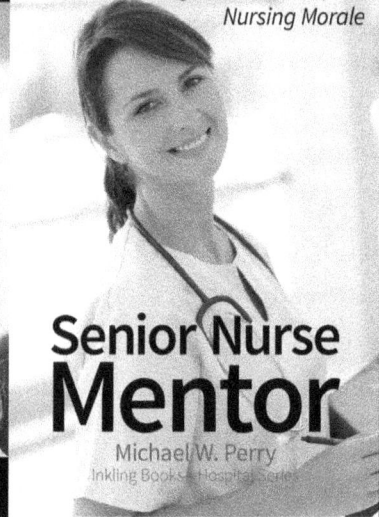

Senior Nurse
Mentor
Michael W. Perry
Inkling Books Hospital Series

HOSPITAL GOWNS

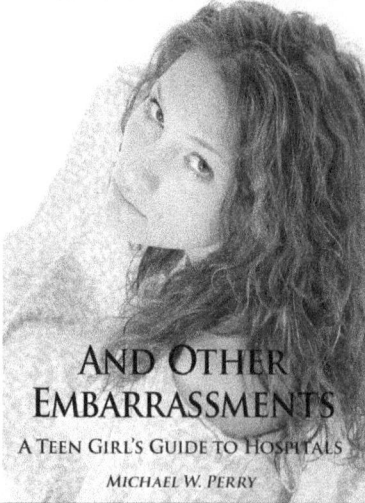

AND OTHER
EMBARRASSMENTS
A TEEN GIRL'S GUIDE TO HOSPITALS
MICHAEL W. PERRY

EMBARRASS LESS

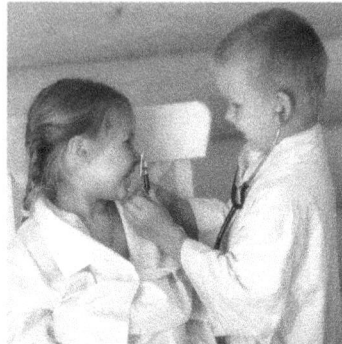

A PRACTICAL GUIDE FOR DOCTORS,
NURSES, STUDENTS AND HOSPITALS
MICHAEL W. PERRY
INKLING BOOKS HOSPITAL SERIES

1. LEUKEMIC CHILDREN

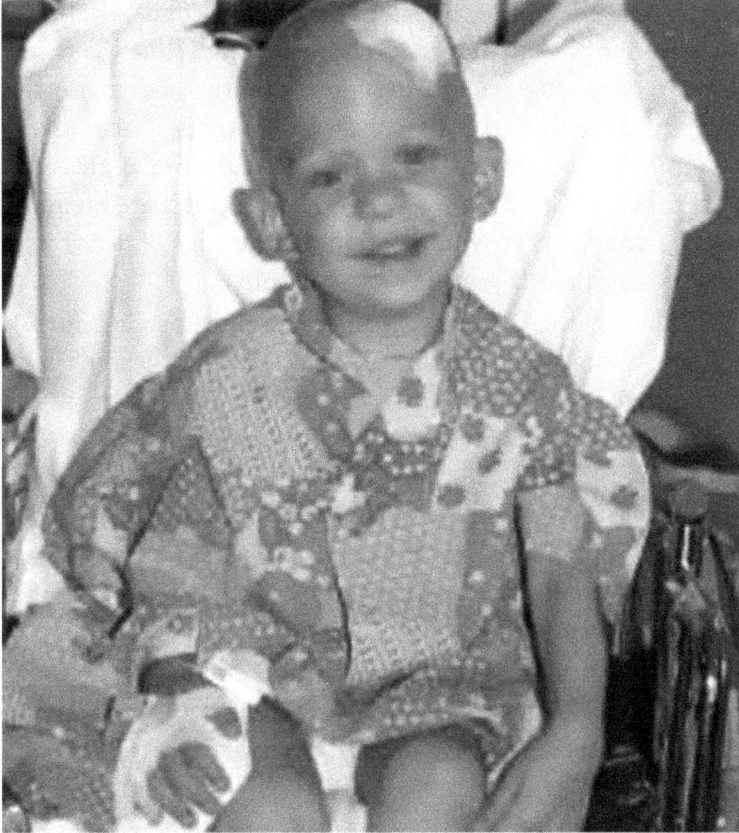

That's a great picture isn't it? The experiences that inspired this book began with children much like him. They're perhaps the only hospitalized patients who don't find their stay embarrassing. That's why I've written this book. Hospitals need to become less embarrassing. Everyone will be happier when they do.

From all the IV pokes he's endured, it's obvious he was one of my earliest patients. Notice the site on the top of his head and the current one in his right hand. Before that, he almost certainly had at least two more, one at each elbow. Those were the easiest, so we started with them, although they didn't last long. A few weeks into being treated for childhood leukemia, he has endured at least four pokes along with daily blood draws. Fortunately, that misery would soon end, as our Hem-Onc unit became one of the first to use central lines routinely for pediatric oncology.

Of course the pokes, which are over in seconds, are nothing in comparison to the chemotherapy we dealt out. This was the era that *The Emperor of All Maladies* describes bluntly, one where the temporary successes of various cancer treatments, "were like truces declared in the battle—signs, merely, that a more aggressive attack was necessary. The allure of deploying a full armamentarium of cytotoxic drugs—of driving the body to the edge of death to rid it of its malignant innards—was still irresistible."

We did just that. In our efforts to cure, we pushed our wonderful little children to the brink of death. No, we weren't fools. We realized that some were put at more risk by our treatments than by their cancers. We knew that too little treatment for one might be too much for another. But how were our specialists to know? Childhood leukemia moves incredibly fast. Our children could not wait for a genetic understanding of their cancer. The result was aggressive treatment followed by an equally aggressive response to terrifyingly low blood counts. Our kids went through a lot, and we were why.

How did I find myself in such a situation? Not by the usual path. My college major was in engineering rather than medicine or nursing. Therein lies a tale that I explain better in *My Nights with Leukemia*. Here's a snapshot.

I was working for a small energy-management company that was spiraling into bankruptcy. On impulse, I took an Emergency Medical Technician (EMT) course at a community college. I thought of volunteering as a mountain search and rescue medic. When the company laid me off, I looked for work. A friend suggested I apply for what today would be a nurse tech position at a nearby children's hospital. It'd be a change, I thought, and would use that EMT training. I was accepted for nights (11 p.m. to 7 a.m.) on a medical unit caring for kids from one to nine.

Orientation on days was terrible. The kids were fun, but few stayed long enough for me to know them. Most work was dull and repetitive, like being a maid in a hotel. I'm not suited for that. As my month-long orientation wrapped up, I wondered if nights would be different enough to make the work bearable. I knew I did not want to work on Hem-Onc, which at that time was one of the medical unit's three clusters of rooms and off-limits to other staff. One look at those children, pale and emaciated with only a few wisps of hair, was enough to tell me to stay away.

Then came my first night shift, and I found I'd been hired specifically to work Hem-Onc alongside a nurse. Only later did I realize that placing me in such a difficult position *with no task-specific orientation* warned of an administrative shift from training nurses well to condemning them for mistakes made due to poor training. I was fortunate. Three experienced nurses mentored me marvelously. If I'd been hired later, I would not have learned nearly as much. They turned a newly minted EMT into a qualified Hem-Onc nurse tech.

My transformation from fearing to liking came so suddenly, I don't recall the specifics. Despite the emotional risks, I found meaning in caring for seven extremely sick children, almost all with leukemia. The very severity of their illness made it easy to be good. When you place personal ease on one side of a scale and "a child dies" on the other, decisions are easy.

Between the chemotherapy and a terrible prognosis, the work was grim. At that time the cure rate for the most common childhood leukemia (ALL) was 70 percent, a remarkable improvement over two decades earlier. But that still meant that on most nights two of my young patients—their average age was four—would eventually die. Adding to that stress, the nurse I worked with spent her time managing complex IVs. My job was to watch over those children and sound the alarm if one got into trouble. If I failed, even a few hours of delay might mean a child's death.

I was mystified by how smoothly I slid into the work, particularly the sense that I was meant to be there. How can that be? Nothing in my education or experience prepared me for it—or so I thought. Early on, I understood one reason I felt at home there. I enjoyed caring for the same children night after night. What might scare away others, the fear of losing a child they liked, drove me all the harder. For sixteen months I never relaxed. A single second might contain the fleeting thought that warned me a child was in trouble. A child's mental status often altered before the numbers went bad.

Only recently, as some long-forgotten memories came back, did I realize there was another reason I took naturally to the work. When I was the age of my young patients, I watched a cousin named Beth waste away and die. She had cystic fibrosis, but her appearance in those last months was much like the patients I was caring for. I thought the world of Hem-Onc was new to me. It wasn't.

With those returning memories, I recalled the intense fury I felt as a young child. I was angry, but didn't know where to direct my anger. I wanted to keep Beth from dying, but was powerless. Those feelings lay submerged for three decades until, without my being aware, they resurfaced when I began to care for those children. What I hadn't been able to do for her, I could do for them. I could give them a chance at life. Even their deaths did not frighten me. I'd been through her death. I could go through those dark hours again. None of that was conscious, but it was real.

Later, I would realize that my lack of the usual preparatory schooling shaped how I approached work. Having never attended medical or nursing school, I had no packaged answers for the problems I faced. Engineers build things. They aren't taught that it is acceptable to inflict pain on sweet children. I had to come up with solutions that worked for me. I accepted that most of what those kids went through was necessary, but I never conceded an inch more. I saw their suffering as a great evil to be hated with all the fury I could muster. Any time I could shove back, I did, no matter how small the push. At times that felt like spitting into a hurricane. But I knew that as long as I spit, that evil had not won.

The brutal hammer blows of their chemotherapy typically surfaced around one or two a.m., when our drugs hit toxic levels. Their bodies knew that, and they vomited in a futile effort to rid themselves of the poison we were pouring into their veins, I'd stay with them, holding a small bucket. That was the pitifully little I could do. I didn't want a child to associate his parents with that pain. Parents felt the same. None ever insisted on taking my place. But I also knew that meant the child might associate that pain with me. Next to a mistake that might kill a child, that bothered me the most.

"Would they blame me for this?," I asked in those early weeks. To my amazement, they didn't. By some magic, they were able to separate their sickness from their treatment. Even more amazingly, I found that they liked and trusted me.

You see that in the wonderful smile on the face to the little boy whose picture opens this chapter. He had a loving grandmother who made a huge difference. Not all our kids were that fortunate. For the first child I cared for who died, an overwhelmed single mother could not stay overnight, so I had to be her substitute, rocking her terrified two-year-old son to sleep. Even worse were three children with cancer who were abandoned to us. No one in their family visited. As staff, we had to make up for their absence. As busy as we were, that never worked well.

I soon discovered that the key to winning the trust of those children was simple. I liked them and did my best to show it. Children have an great sense of who likes them. If you don't, they know it. They even notice when an adult's liking has reservations—such as only liking kids who remain quiet.

Yes, I hated what we were doing and that never altered. I was an outsider, an engineer trained to be objective almost to a fault. Nothing had prepared me for this medical house of horrors. I was making up responses as I went. My efforts to explain those feelings sometimes went astray. The nurses I worked with didn't understand that I wasn't being flippant when I told them, "A hospital is the worst place to be when you're sick." I wasn't downplaying the marvelous ability of modern hospitals to cure even once-fatal illnesses such as childhood leukemia. I was pointing out that the curing often came with an excess of the three ills of hospitalization: pain, hassle, and embarrassment. Those are what made hospitalization bad.

After sixteen months of working nights with three different groups of nurses, I would transfer to day shift on Teens, the unit that cared for most patients from ten and up. In the next chapter will take a brief look at teen embarrassment to lay the foundation for what comes later. Keep in mind that my experiences on Hem-Onc shaped how I would react to later events on Teens. I'd deal with embarrassment on Teens much like I'd handled pain on Hem-Onc.

2. Embarrassed Teens

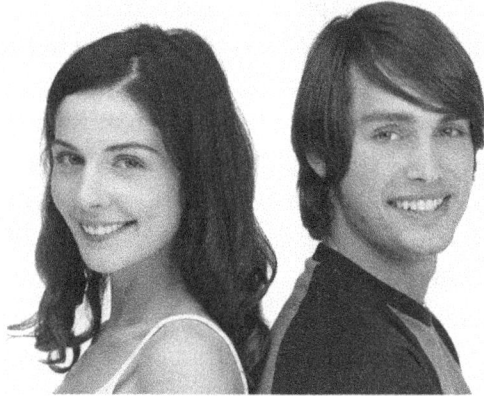

While I wrestled with the misery we afflicted on small children, I would occasionally face a different issue—the embarrassment felt by teens who overflowed, typically for a single night, onto our unit. Each in turn helped me to understand just a little better how they felt. Thanks to them, I came to realize that embarrassment mattered as much to teens as pain did to children. A visit to any high school will demonstrate just how much teens fear it. When a teen says, "I could die...," he or she is almost always referring to embarrassment.

The issues with embarrassment that teens brought to Hem-Onc would prepare me for what I would face when I transferred to care for them full-time. *My Nights with Leukemia* focuses on my experience with small kids with leukemia. This book centers on teens and the embarrassment they felt. Both are written primarily for healthcare professionals, but should benefit anyone.

Now for a little psychology, at its heart, like pain, embarrassment is a stress and patients respond accordingly. Unfortunately, grown adults are not transparent enough to serve as reliable guides. They've learned what is expected of them and act accordingly, often concealing their true feelings. I do that myself.

That's why describing my experience with these teens matters. As any parent can attest, teens conceal their feelings poorly. So if you'd like an explanation for why I feel qualified to write this book, that's it. I learned a lot about teen responses to embarrassment and that experience can tell us what's going on in the minds of others, including adults of both sexes and all ages.

This book represents my effort to translate their responses into useful ideas. There's certainly a need. While I was researching the first book in this hospital series, a guide for hospitalized teen girls called *Hospital Gowns and Other Embarrassments*, a research librarian at one of the country's top health science schools and I spent 45 minutes searching medical and nursing databases for anything on patient embarrassment. We tried every term we could imagine and drew a blank. The closest was an article on "integrity issues" for Iranian women in Iranian hospitals. Since then I've heard of a Canadian study which found—to no one's surprise—that many hospitalized patients did not need the embarrassing gowns they were expected to wear. They could have been cared for just as easily with clothing that left them feeling more comfortable. That limited research is one reason why I've written this. I want to break down the wall of silence and encourage others better placed than I to do more formal research. This area has been neglected far too long.

There was another benefit to my experience. That was the peculiar position I found myself in. As I've already mentioned, on Hem-Onc the stresses on our children were a result of the miseries we deliberately inflicted on them. I hoped those children would make a distinction between me and those miseries. To my relief, they did. When I started on Teens. I faced a different problem. Pain was not that great an issue with teenagers. They typically take it stoically, realizing it's necessary. The more important issue was embarrassment in a broad sense, and that we had in abundance.

One reason was the type of care we specialized in. We did so many orthopedic surgeries, at that time "Orthopedic" was a part of the hospital's name. After those surgeries, our teen boys and girls were heavily dependent on staff, creating an abundance of embarrassing situations. I'll explain that in more detail later, but for now keep in mind that for the boys their embarrassment centered on the fact that the rest of our nursing staff was female. I could do little to correct that. For our girls, however, as the only man on our nursing staff, I was the totality of their problem. If they became embarrassed, I was the cause. I couldn't evade that fact.

But there was an upside. If I was the cause, then I could also be the answer. All I need do was change what I did. Fortunately for me, the feelings of those girls proved so marvelously transparent. I could know, often in an instant, if what I was doing worked or didn't. That let me discover practical ways to ease their minds. Much of this book is based on what they taught me. To them and to their patience with my blunders, I owe a great thanks.

There's another benefit that flows from my particular circumstances. I'm skeptical that the radical emotional differences I found between teen boys and teen girls exist in every hospital. That seems unlikely. But whether it does or not, that wide gap is helpful. Patients respond to stresses such as embarrassment differently, and those differences must taken into account. In the boys and girls I cared for, I saw those differences starkly illustrated. The boys reacted one way, and the girls in another. Both matter, irrespective of sex, because in any hospital situation, patients—whatever their sex and age—will tend toward one or the other of these two extremes. It's wired into our natures. Keep that in mind with your patients.

When I went into a room with teen boys recovering from major surgeries, I found withdrawal and no more than grudging compliance. Psychologists call that a fight-or-flight response. They couldn't fight, so they fled. In this book you'll read about the frustrations that caused me. "These are guys like me," I thought over and over again during those ten months, "Why can't they lighten up when I'm doing their care?" I knew one reason. Because at any moment one of our pretty nurses might burst in, leaving them flustered.

In contrast, when I went into a room with teen girls, I found them eager to cooperate. That's a tend-and-befriend response. With them, I was soon telling myself, "These girls are wonderful. They make my work much easier." I liked to know my patients, so their warm response made up for the frustrations I felt with the boys.

More than once I asked myself why those guys couldn't be more like the girls. From the girls, I learned much. From the guys I found myself slamming into a stone wall, learning little. Whatever I did was met with resistance. Looking back, I now understand some what I should have known then. I should have eased their frustrations and found ways to shift their response from an unproductive fight-or-flight response to a more helpful tend-and-befriend. That would have helped. I did have a few guys—typically experienced patients with major disabilities or long-term illnesses—who weren't withdrawn. With them, our relationship went far better. That's something you might consider when you have patients of either sex who are locked into a fight-or-flight response. Get them to focus on befriending staff and other patients instead of resisting treatment. Both they and you will be happier.

Praise for those boys would have helped too. As I will explain in more detail later, these guys wanted to impress their nurses. Feeling unable to accomplish that like most teen guys do—by showing off— they withdrew. What could those boys be praised for? I've pondered that, and at first it seemed insolvable. How do you praise a guy who is lying helpless in bed with one leg in traction? He can do almost nothing for himself. Then it came to me. You praise him for what he was doing before he needed that surgery—maybe even for whatever act of male adolescent craziness landed him in the hospital. Everyone is good at something. Find out what it is and speak well of it. Then these guys might lighten up.

Vividness is an added benefit of the descriptions you'll find here. Although you may not find yourself in a similar situation to mine, there's an advantage to looking at adolescents. Teens are experts at creating drama. There is no need for me to embellish what happened. Every account you will read is as accurate as I can recall. But these accounts are rendered all the more colorful by the strong passions felt by my young patients, much as ordinary sunlight is transformed by a stained glass window. Vivid contrasts then make for great writing. G. K. Chesterton defended Charles Dickens against critics that way.

But while these are real characters they are real characters lit up with the colors of youth and passion. They are real people romantically felt; that is to say, they are real people felt as real people feel them. They are exaggerated, like all Dickens's figures: but they are not exaggerated as personalities are exaggerated by an artist; they are exaggerated as personalities are exaggerated by their own friends and enemies. The strong souls are seen through the glorious haze of the emotions that strong souls really create.

That's what I hope you'll discover here. My patient's zest for their young lives, as well as my strong desire to care for them, transformed events that might otherwise seem sheer drudgery—bedpans, linen sheets, and even vomit—into something of great interest. It was they who made this a joy to write. I hope you find them as fascinating as I did.

I also hope you'll sympathize with these teens as they struggle, tossed about in a sea of troubles at such a young age. Little twelve-year-old Tina's desperate battle to live at whatever the cost to herself carries an important message, as does Christy's gentleness as she lay dying with a mother gone mad. Min's fears, as well as the swelteringly hot room of the post-op girls, raise issues about patient care that need answering. This book is not about the dull and dreary mechanics of hospital care. That's merely incidental. It's a drama, with real people going through some of the most difficult experiences of their lives. I did not find writing it boring. I hope you find reading it fascinating.

Judging by the response to *Hospital Gowns*, many readers will be delighted that this book brings up a topic that's long needed discussing. But there are likely to be some who feel I treat embarrassment wrongly. I'll address their concerns here.

Some will suggest that I treat embarrassment far too seriously. Patients, they will claim, readily adapt to embarrassment. Look, they say, at how rarely they speak up and protest. Not so, I say, and I give examples, including young Min, trapped in her body cast, who said nothing but was terrified by my male presence. We should not mistake patients who are intimidated into silence with comfortable patients. Patients aren't happy simply because they don't scream in protest. Silence can be an indication of fear.

On the other hand, some may insist that what I say is of little importance. A little embarrassment, they will point out, is nothing in comparison to dying. I agree that's true, and I've had my share of the latter. But we must place "unnecessary" in front of "embarrassing." Medical treatment does involve embarrassment much as it does pain, on that we agree. But that does not mean it has to be as embarrassing as it often is. That's one of the central points of this book. Embarrassment can and should be handled better. That's not impossible or even that hard. It simply means making it a priority and learning by experience what works and what doesn't.

Interestingly, all the books in my hospital series began with a failure take embarrassment seriously. I saw a news story about an elderly British woman who wanted the National Health Service to send her only women home-care workers—a reasonable request. A callous NHS bureaucracy turned her down. Angry about that, I recalled my own experiences with similar issues. I realized in the flood of memories that followed that I had the makings of several books, including this one.

I may also get flack from the opposite direction. Some will be upset by the casualness and even humor I find in some situations. I talk too casually, they will complain, about girls recovering from back surgeries who roll on their sides, with the backs of their gowns flopping open. They forget that those girls and I had an unspoken agreement. They could roll on their sides to find comfort in a miserably hot room. In return, I would turn away quickly and never stare. There's no reason to get upset. Given the circumstances, that worked well enough. It certainly worked better than what happened with our post-op boys in the same situation. Their zeal to remain covered up in the presence of nurses left them hot and miserable.

Finally, I hope that the sheer likability of my young patients, so refreshingly young and filled with a zest for life, will encourage you to sympathize with the issues faced by your patients, whatever their circumstances. What's true for a shy Maria, a desperate Tina, a gentle Christy, and an overwhelmed Pala, may also be true for your patients, including the grumpiest oldster.

Next, we look at my first two encounters with embarrassment, and how I responded. Neither went well, but my responses will improve, that I promise. I wasn't always as stupid as I seemed then. Telling my tale chronologically does have an advantage. You can learn along with me.

3. INNOCENT MARIA

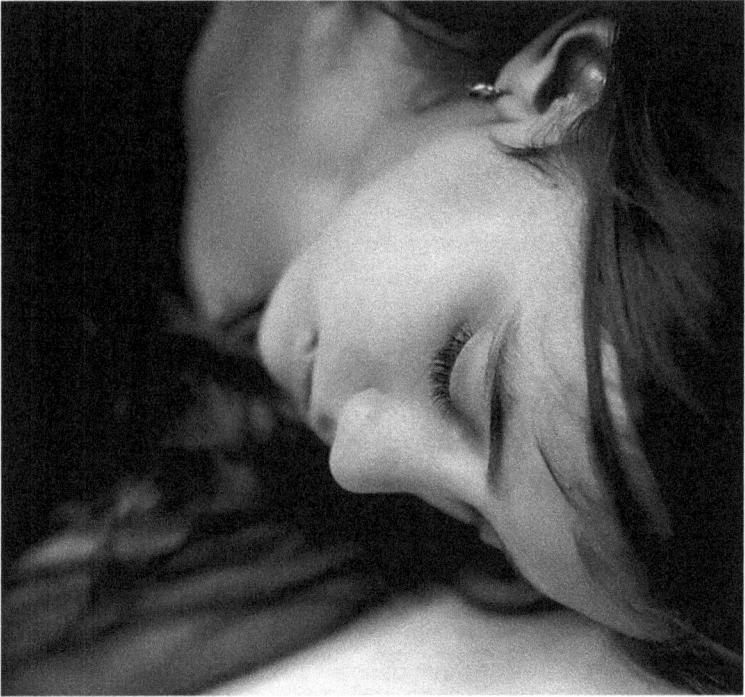

One night, the hospital floated me to Teens, leaving me unhappy. I liked Hem-Onc kids and, thanks to my growing expertise, I floated only when Cala—the third-year nursing student who shared my position—was also working. On Teens, I'd typically spend but a single night with numerous patients I never got to know, much like working in a hotel.

Around two in the morning, a mother came from one of the private rooms, saw me, and rushed up in a panic. Could I please help, she asked, explaining that her daughter's bedpan was about to overflow. The nurse I was working with wasn't in sight. With seventeen patients demanding her attention, she rarely was.

I went into the darkened room. The mother was right. The bedpan of a girl we'll call Amy was filled within a quarter of an inch of the top. Some idiot had left a child's bedpan in the room of a seventeen-year-old girl whose after-chemotherapy IV was running fast. Not knowing any better, the mother had used it.

Slowly, ever so slowly, I inched that bedpan from underneath Amy. As I did, I heard her sobbing quietly. This must be humiliating, I thought. But alas, as well-trained in hospital culture as I was, I made little of that. "I'm doing my best," I thought, "even though that makes it harder. I'm doing this from the side, so all I can see are her hips. Besides, if this bedpan spills, that'll mean a linen change, which will be even more embarrassing."

Excuses, excuses, excuses—hospitals are filled with them. We're doing our best, the staff say, much like I told myself that night. Maybe we are. But it's also possible we can improve what we do. In fact, knowing how to deal with embarrassment may actually *improve* care. Embarrassment interferes with good medicine much like pain does. Staff shy away from procedures they'd otherwise follow because of pain or embarrassment. Patients hesitate to report problems, knowing either may follow. A brilliant Google software developer told me she'd delayed much needed medical care from a fear of embarrassment. That's not good.

But notice that this book's title is *Embarrass Less* rather than "Embarrass Not." I'm well aware that a hospital isn't a five-star hotel. Embarrassment cannot be completely eliminated. But the suggestions you'll find here have been tested and do work. They will leave patients happier. Keep in mind a critical fact. When embarrassment drops below a certain level, patient anxiety often disappears altogether. Patients feel in control and secure. In practice, *less* embarrassment may mean *no* embarrassment. I saw that over and over. That's encouraging. With just a little effort, you can turn morose patients into happy ones.

In the end, I handled Amy poorly. My excuse is that she was the first such situation I faced, and none of my training had prepared me. Lack of awareness and insufficient training will come up again and again. That needs to change. Embarrassment is serious and should be treated as such. Staff need to be taught to handle it. They need to be rewarded when they handle it well and to have people they can turn to for advice when they have questions. Being too embarrassed to discuss embarrassment makes no sense.

Normally, when I did something badly, I wouldn't rest until I'd found a better way. When I first began, one nurse helped me with that more than any other. She was careful and taught me to be the same. That's good, particularly on Hem-Onc. But there was one area in which we disagreed.

We totaled fluids for our patients at 6 a.m. She did IVs, while I did voids. Often, we'd have a child who'd come in the day before and whose follow-up chemotherapy hadn't begun. There was no IV and no voids. I believed that, "nothing in means nothing out is fine." She believed, and I quote, "Every kid pees on my shift."

As you see, we differed in the importance we attached to hassle versus caution. The real issue was timing. Getting fluid out for those 6 a.m. totals meant waking a child. Since it might be weeks before that child got another full night's sleep, I hated that. With that nurse, I gritted my teeth and woke the child. With other nurses I skipped the void, until I realized there was another factor that I needed to take into account.

Bitter about their lives, two of Hem-Onc's day nurses were nasty with our younger night nurses. "What if they squawk about my zero total?," I thought, "I might be forced to make those 6 a.m. voids." Ah, but I saw an answer. When day shift arrived, noisy as stampeding buffaloes, our children woke up. That could not be helped. Then I could get that void. Should those ill-tempered nurses complain about that zero total, I could point to the 7 a.m. void and say, "See, nothing is wrong." From that, I'd learned something important, which was how to reconcile conflicting expectations. I'd use that later with teen embarrassment.

Unfortunately, what happened with Amy did not force me to think about solutions. I learned nothing, because I believed I'd done my best. Besides, my thoughts were occupied with those little kids fighting to live. I would have probably forgotten this incident, but for what happened one night with the shy and innocent Maria.

Most nights, work on Hem-Onc was steady and predictable. We worked hard to achieve that because an emergency might mean a child died. Given how fragile our patients were, it was far better to prevent a crisis than to deal with one. When a child's platelet count approached the danger zone, we gave platelets. When one spiked a temperature, we started broad-spectrum antibiotics. When a child needed extra attention, we adjusted our schedules to free up time. We took no chances.

This night was unusual in that our work was actually slow. Aware of that by some mysterious power, Admitting assigned two girls to us and put them in a little-used room next to Hem-Onc. One was five and in only to have her temperature checked every two hours. The other, although she seemed in no pain, would be getting an emergency appendectomy the next day.

Maria, the surgery patient, was fourteen. She was Hispanic, cute and petite, with dark hair and eyes, so she looked much like the stock photo at the start of this chapter. She was apprehensive about what was probably her first surgery. Since we had time to spare, her nurse and I did our best to calm her.

About midnight, I was with the five-year-old when Maria asked the nurse for a bedpan. The nurse responded all too professionally, "Mike will take care of that," and hurried away. In one sense she was right. Bedpans, urinals, and diapers were my responsibility not hers.

Alas, shy Maria wanted a female nurse but was stuck with me, a guy with a manly beard. What was she to do? Her plight is why in *Hospital Gowns* I stress to teen girls that they should not expect staff women, either doctors or nurses, to spare them from embarrassment. Often they won't. Later, I'll explain why.

Here's some background for those who've not worked in hospitals. Medical units are all about fluids. Patients are often on IVs, so the staff focuses on fluids coming in and out. Hem-Onc was that multiplied by ten. Our kids had two or sometimes three IV pumps running around the clock, with their treatments constantly changing. They received antibiotics, blood products, chemotherapy, nutrition, pain medications, and even nasty anti-viral drugs. That's why the nurses complained that they spent more time with IVs than with patients. My gripe was that I spent my time doing "pee-pee checks." I monitored and recorded the volume and often PH of urine for each child. As I mentioned, near the end of each shift, fluids out needed to be almost the same as fluids in. The work was dull and repetitive but necessary. I knew it mattered, so I endured the drudgery.

That's why, when I went to take care of Maria's bedpan, I was like a robot, doing what I'd done hundreds of times before with little kids. I pulled down her sheet, flipped up her gown, and pulled down her undies all in one quick motion. I'd done that so many times, I didn't need to look.

Matters would have stood at that but for something different which happened that night. Hem-Onc nights almost never received new admissions. Our patients were scheduled well in advance. When one left, another came within a few hours, typically during the day. But because Maria had arrived late in the evening, the previous shift had not written a nursing assessment. That delighted the newly graduated nurse I was working with. After her assessment was done, she asked me to read it and give my opinion.

What she'd written was good, but one comment ticked me off. She wrote that Maria "denies recent sexual activity." Yes, I knew that was mere boilerplate, placed there because Maria's complaints were abdominal and at least theoretically might have been the result of a sexually transmitted disease. But Maria was a such an innocent girl—something the nurse knew as well as I—that I became angry. I considered stomping up to her, pointing to that phrase, and saying, "With that 'denies recent,' you insult Maria. You make her sound like an out-of-work prostitute."

Then the incongruity of what I'd be doing struck me. Maria would never see what her nurse had written. But she had seen me come up and treat her like I would treat a small boy who'd wet his pants. I was a far worse offender than this nurse. Outside the hospital, what I'd done might have gotten me arrested.

Looking back, it took seeing my own hypocrisy to make me aware that nothing in my training or that of my nurse made either of us aware that we shouldn't be treating a fourteen-year-old girl like a four-year-old boy, particularly when there was such an easy choice between caregivers. Slow as that night was, the nurse could have easily taken care of that bedpan. The fact that she did not illustrates a strange but common attitude in hospitals that I call "staff are not male or female." It's strange because patients rarely share that feeling. It's common because it simplifies decision making. The sex of the caregiver and patient are treated as irrelevant. That brings up a major point of this book. Staff *are* male and female. They need to be regarded as such. Recognizing that is not the end of the world.

Fortunately, no harm followed. Maria was as trusting as she was sweet and must have regarded what happened as yet another inexplicable part of being hospitalized. That night, she continued to be friendly with both of us. But she should have been treated better than that. Unlike with Amy, this time I realized I had made a mistake. I asked myself what I should have done differently.

First comes a disclaimer. Keep mind that at this point the complications of caring for teen girls such as Maria weren't my focus. They came to us perhaps once every six weeks when there wasn't a bed on Teens and then typically only as one girl for one night. In fact, they were so rare that I never noticed that they were almost always girls. The "almost" explains why. The first teen I cared for was a fourteen-year-old boy getting an early pediatric bone marrow transplant. That meant I didn't notice the pattern with normal overflows. Looking back, Admissions must have sent the teen boys to the surgery unit, one floor up, and sent us the girls. Also, most of these girls were well enough—typically just before or after ordinary surgeries—that they needed little attention. We simply gave them a bed for the night. Busy as we were, they were easy to ignore.

No, what mattered to me were the kids from one to nine that I cared for every night. Could I learn something from my clumsy treatment of Maria to benefit them? Our younger kids, I realized, were not an issue. Nothing embarrassed them. Being hospitalized was like "playing doctor." Their bewitching innocence is where I got the idea for this book's cover. I wanted a light-hearted cover to balance out a book that must be serious at times. If anything, those little children may have wondered why we weren't giving them 'owies' on their little bottoms like their family doctor did. Although missing their parents, most were happy enough with us. I didn't need to change how they were treated.

But when I thought of our older kids, something did come to mind. About six or seven, the kids on Hem-Onc began to behave differently. Rather than use a call light or ask for a urinal or bedpan when I came into their room, they'd wake their parents. When I appeared later, a urinal or bedpan would be waiting by the sink for those endless pee-pee checks. In the past, I'd simply enjoyed that as one less thing to do. Now I saw it differently. Those six-and-up kids were developing a sense of modesty, probably by imitating adults. Since it seemed the same for boys and girls, it wasn't sexually tinged.

There was another factor I discovered when I asked an administrator why children were transferred from our medical unit to Teens at ten rather than puberty. She explained that at about ten, boys and girls become curious about the opposite sex. That made keeping them in a multi-bed room awkward. Modesty at six, curiosity at ten, and budding sexuality at twelve was the progression. Age matters, I realized, so I began to take it into account.

Another factor complicated matters. If all children six and up had parents staying with them, modesty would not have been an issue. But some parents of older children with leukemia could not stay overnight, and the larger medical unit where I also worked had multi-bed rooms with no space for parents to sleep. I needed some practical way to handle the modesty of kids six and up when parents weren't around.

The answer proved easy. Almost all these kids wore underpants, so I adopted the simple expedient of slipping a bedpan in place first, then slipping down their cartoon-character undies beneath their gowns. I also realized that was how I should have treated Maria. That only took a few seconds longer and was far less embarrassing. Only when I transferred to Teens did I discover that this new technique had a serious flaw. More on that later.

Next, we'll look at a girl who had a no-nonsense way of dealing with embarrassment. Her response wasn't just rare. As sensible as it might appear, it was the only such response I saw during my entire 26 months at the hospital. Later, we'll see why that matters.

4. GRUMPY BARB

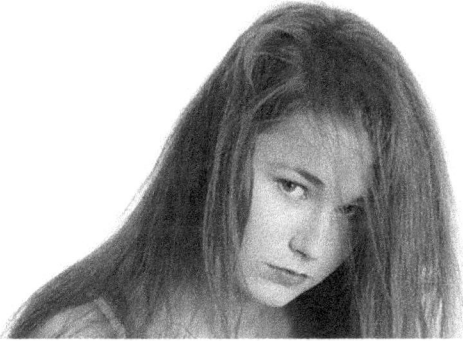

Like them or not, grumpy patients can teach us much about what other patients may be feeling but not saying. In this chapter we will look at a most exceptional girl. Outliers like her help us to establish boundaries. She did something no other girl I cared for ever did—she flatly refused to be embarrassed. For that, she deserves all the praise I bestow on her in *Hospital Gowns*.

I was working with ordinary medical kids that night. A little after midnight, we got a call from the ER. They had a teen girl for us. I went to transport her and found I was early. The front desk clerk told me she was in an exam room with a resident. I went in and found an abundance of loveliness. Barb, a pretty, fifteen-year-old, was talking with Dr. Lovely, our loveliest and, in my estimation, smartest woman resident.

How did I know Dr. Lovely was smart? Easy, because she asked me for advice and took my suggestions. I liked the residents who did that. They knew nursing staff had more hands-on experience than they. In contrast, the less talented seemed terrified that someone might challenge their judgment. They made mistakes they'd could have avoided had they only listened.

Barb had a sunburn that was painful but not dangerous. As I entered, Dr. Lovely was offering to apply a lotion to ease the inflammation. That's when a potentially embarrassing situation arose that I saw all too often. The sunburn was on the girl's chest or, to be more precise, her breasts. Since I wasn't needed, I decided leave, but I hated those embarrass-or-flee situations. Whatever I did felt wrong. Staying when I wasn't needed made me feel like a pervert. Slinking away made me feel like a recovering pervert. Something should be done to make those exits less awkward for opposite-sex staff. In this case, perhaps Dr. Lovely might have said, "After this gentleman leaves, I will...." That would have been my exit cue. I'd have felt better, and this girl would have felt more assured.

A few minutes later, Barb came out, and I walked her to the medical unit. When we arrived, I began filling out the admission paperwork. At one point, I needed her weight, so I asked her to stand on a scale. Only then, as she faced away, did I realized why she was clutching her blanket so tightly. Her bare arms, shoulders, and back spoke clearly. Someone in the ER had taken away her blouse and not bothered to returned it. Without that blanket, she'd be topless.

Since I didn't know the blanket's weight, I suggested she put it down while facing away from me. That's when she uttered those momentous but ever-so-rare words, "No way." That wasn't a problem. I took her weight with the blanket and subtracted a couple of kilograms. In her case, accuracy mattered little.

Why, I asked myself as I wrote this book, did she—alone among all the girls I cared for—refuse to do something that wasn't actually embarrassing, when so many others submitted to genuine embarrassment without a word of protest? There are a couple of reasons.

First, most of the girls I cared for were seriously sick and eager to cooperate with those who would get them well. Barb was clearly ticked off and felt no need to pander to anyone. If I were to reconstruct events, it'd run something like this.

Her face, arms, and back weren't sunburned, nor was the top of her chest above the blanket, so it's not hard to work out what happened. That day Barb had foolishly tried to get a topless tan. She forgot that skin that's never been tanned burns easily. She was now angry at herself for being so stupid. That evening after she went to bed, she discovered that her sunburn made sleep impossible and told her parents. They probably replied with, "You did what?" Then they drove her to our ER, with everyone in the car seething with anger. Since it was after midnight when they arrived, they left her with some pointed "you got yourself into this mess" remarks. That explained why, rather than go home after receiving the ointment, she had to stay overnight.

Barb's troubles did not end there. ER's all-female staff took her blouse and failed to return it, forcing her to clutch that blanket. My request that she lay it down became the final straw, hence her "No way." She'd been pushed enough. She would not go one inch further. In *Hospital Gowns*, I tell readers that her firmness was commendable, but her ticked-off attitude wasn't necessary. Say "no," I tell those girls, but say it nicely. Hospital staff endure enough criticism. They don't need more.

Barb's second reason matters more. Most patients came to us in great need. We were the premier children's hospital for one fourth the land area of the U.S., including Alaska. Many patients needed care only we could provide. They felt they must go along, even with embarrassing situations. They feared their illness more than they feared embarrassment—as if they must choose between the two.

I did my best to counter that fear in *Hospital Gowns*. I stress to my readers—primarily teen girls—that a cheerful, cooperative attitude coupled with a firmness about what they feel uncomfortable about will go over well with nurses. They don't need to be afraid that a "no" to embarrassment will get them put onto some dreadful black list, with words like these: "Ah, I see you refused to be embarrassed earlier today in front of a dozen leering male premed students. That we do not permit. There will be no pain pills for you tonight. You must lie awake, miserable, to consider the error of your ways."

Barb was a notable exception. She was in our hospital only because her parents had dumped her on us. After that lotion was applied, she needed us no more. In a pinch, she could call a friend to pick her up. Even more important, she didn't have to do what I said. She had no reason to care whether I liked her or not.

What should I have done differently? First, I shouldn't have been grumpy about having my work interrupted by an unexpected, middle-of-the night admission. Then I would have been thinking more clearly. Second, I should have been more observant of her situation. Before we left the ER, I should have noticed her missing blouse and had the staff recover it. I needed to learn to never transport a patient without looking for things being left behind. If she'd gotten her blouse back in the ER, she would have been less grouchy.

Note that it took all that on her part—doing something stupid, being in pain, clashing with parents, feeling extremely ticked off, having her blouse taken away, and not needing hospitalization—to get her to say "No way" to being *almost* embarrassed. That should tell us that we need to be gentle about the hidden pressures we put on patients. We need to avoid as much as possible the hidden coercion that comes with hospitalization.

The next girl we discuss illustrates what happens when that isn't done. Tina's desperation became one of my saddest experiences, one made all the worse by the fact that she was my patient for but a single night. I would never see her again.

5. Desperate Tina

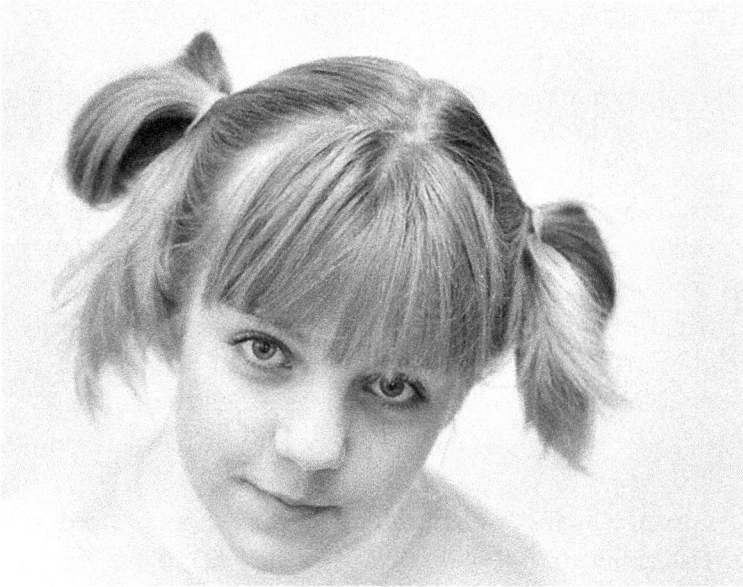

About five a.m., as I was checking on the kids in a multi-bed room, I heard someone move behind a curtain. She was the mother of the slender, twelve-year-old Tina. The girl had wet herself, and her mother had just finished changing her clothes and sheets. I felt doubly guilty. First, because I hadn't checked on Tina since midnight. Second, because I thought I might be responsible for that wetting.

The first guilt was easily dismissed. Tina, who had leukemia, was to start her follow-up chemotherapy the next day. Since Teens didn't have a bed free, she came to us. Because she was no different from when she'd been at home the night before, my orders were to check her at midnight and then leave her alone. That I had done. I hated waking up sick kids even when it was necessary. With her, it wasn't necessary.

I think I understand now why she wet herself. Kids coming in for their first chemotherapy don't grasp how bad it is. Their treatment so closely follows their diagnosis, typically by a couple of days, that they have little time for dread or fear. Subsequent chemotherapies are different. They know what to expect. Despite the added risk, a few of the children I cared for insisted on being drugged into oblivion for their follow-up chemotherapy. In Tina's case, her anxiety must have kept her from sleeping her last few nights at home. Hospitalized and exhausted, she had slept too deeply and wet herself.

My other guilt wasn't so easy to dismiss. Had the fact that she had me, a guy, for her caregiver meant she didn't ask for help when she needed it, fallen back to sleep, and wet herself? That made sense. She was twelve, an age when quickly changing bodies give boys and girls additional reasons for shyness. But as I thought about that, I dismissed the idea as ridiculous. First, as I talked to her mother, she was sitting up in bed making no effort to cover what pitifully little she had on, tiny panties and what her mother might have called a trainer bra. No shyness or modesty there—too little in fact.

Even more telling was how Tina behaved when I responded to her call light at the start of shift. The moment I arrived, she asked for a bedpan, which I pulled from under the bed and placed beneath her. I was about to do the less embarrassing technique I'd adopted after Maria, but she didn't give me a chance. She sat up and handled the situation in the most embarrassing way possible. No other patient ever did that. Her behavior made no sense. "Why did she do that?," I asked myself.

To understand Tina's motivation, keep in mind that patients vary enormously in how they react to learning that they have a fatal disease. Little kids often responded well. With their short attention spans, if nothing hurt at the moment, they were happy. Only if they were dying, something they knew from how their parents were behaving, did some become terrified and need all the support we could give.

Older kids better understood what they faced. Even when they felt healthy, they knew they weren't. Many were quiet and serious, resolved to beat their disease. Dying, they remained much the same, often hiding their fears deep inside.

Working Hem-Onc, I learned to dislike the classic Kübler-Ross model of dying with its five stages: denial, anger, bargaining, depression, and acceptance. That's not just because, as Elisabeth Küber-Ross later admitted, few actually pass through those stages.

What angered me was that she used psychological terms with negative connotations. She saw *denial*, which is but another term for lying. I saw the *courage* to fight. She saw *anger*. I saw a *justified fury* at the unfairness of life. You get my point. Küber-Ross wanted to hurry the dying along to her only legitimate stage, *acceptance*. I saw more varied responses and regarded each as legitimate. I made an effort to understand and respect every response.

For instance, I saw small children display remarkable courage. Pauline was about four and had severe cystic fibrosis. She developed a pneumonia that no antibiotic could treat. Dying children, whatever the reason, were often sent to Hem-Onc. She came with her doctors predicting she had but two days to live. After four days, she still clung to life, barely conscious of what was happening around her. Her parents decided she was refusing to die in a hospital and insisted on taking her home. They were right. Ten minutes after arriving at the home she loved, Pauline ended her long struggle. She died, but she did so at the time and place of her choosing.

Others seemed to despair from the start. I remember Kimberly as a pretty, eight-year-old with beautiful, light-brown hair. With her good-looks and charm, she'd always gotten what she wanted, but not this time. She had AML, the bad leukemia. The disease was cruel and relentless. Our chemotherapy caused her lovely hair to fall out, and she never went home. Her remission was so fleeting, her first visit became her last. To the very end, she remained lost and bewildered. That was terribly sad.

The girl we're discussing here, Tina, had her own response to her illness. Although she was my patient only for that night, I knew kids with leukemia well enough to see she was exceptional. Like all our patients, she wanted to live. But while most kids relaxed a bit during their treatments, trusting our skills and good intentions, I sensed her desperation, meaning "a state of despair, typically one that results in rash or extreme behavior." How she handled that bedpan was rash and extreme. Why did she do that, I wondered, particularly with a guy she'd met only seconds before?

Now I understand. The key lies in her quickness. "See," she was saying, "I'm making it easy for you. I'm taking up as little of your time as I can. I'm doing everything possible for myself. Now please,

please, please save my life." Shoving aside her modesty was how her desperation expressed itself. That made me want to cry.

Had she been young enough to be one of Hem-Onc's patients, she need do nothing to receive the best care I could give. She could be grumpy and uncooperative. I'd remind myself that she had much to be unhappy about. Saving seconds with bedpans wasn't important. Whatever time she required, I would find, giving up breaks and making the most of every moment. I regularly did that for frightened kids who needed to be rocked to sleep. I would do that for her. That's why she was such a tragedy. Her fears were needless.

How should we see Tina's desperation? First, she is best understood as being in the opposite situation to Barb in the previous chapter. All Barb had was a mere sunburn. She'd didn't need us. She certainly didn't need me. As ticked off as she was, I did not matter. That was why she could say, "No way."

Tina was not like that. She had an illness that's invariably fatal without sophisticated treatment, and our hospital was the best place to get that treatment over a multi-state region. She needed us, and that night she needed me as her primary caregiver. Tina was a particularly sensitive girl who was absolutely terrified of dying. She was willing to do anything. That's why she was desperate to please, even in ways that made no sense. That was where our failure lay. We should have offered her more assurance. In the end, the responsibility lay with us.

Months later, after I transferred to Teens, I saw where the problem lay. The distinction came with how leukemia was treated on the two units. Younger kids were handled by our special seven-bed cluster. We were trained for that and knew we were doing uniquely important work. That's why I wanted to work there. Every night when I went to work, I told myself, "You're caring for children who might die. Treat them kindly and watch them carefully."

On their tenth birthday—literally in the case of one sweet girl— leukemia patients were transferred from Hem-Onc to the catch-all Teens. There every imaginable aliment was handled, including medical, surgical and psychiatric. The only exceptions were when a teen required an ICU, Rehab, or locked psychiatric unit.

As a result, working with teens meant being surrounded by an excess of tragedy. In other books, I tell readers that I was not trying to make them sad when I described my teen patients, that I was just stating things as they were. We were a top-of-the-line children's hospital, one of the best in the country. For younger kids, we treated a wide variety of aliments from not serious to extremely serious. Since we specialized in children, physicians and other hospitals often felt better referring their younger patients to us even when those children weren't that sick. We also provided free care for those whose parents could not pay.

Teens were different. Since teens are almost adults, local hospitals could care for their ordinary illnesses. That meant our teen patients were typically much sicker. You see that in the numbers. We had three units for children from birth to nine. The first took care of babies until age one. Its staff were great, but when I floated there, I fretted about patients who could cry but not point to where it hurt. The second, where I worked, cared for medical patients from one to nine. Often that meant IVs for infections, but it was primarily a catch-all for non-surgical children. The third took care of children from one to nine who were getting surgery. Used to the round-the-clock demands of Hem-Onc, when I floated there I was bored by surgery patients who slept through the night. That left but one unit, Teens, for almost all patients from ten to about twenty. Its fewer patients tended to be much sicker.

With so much tragedy on Teens, its hard-pressed staff suffered from *compassionate overload*. As I found out when I transferred there, patients needed more emotionally than we had to give. Some lost out, and to my frustration that was often those with leukemia. At admission, they were neglected because someone newly diagnosed with leukemia doesn't usually look sick. After chemotherapy had done its worst, they often got less attention for the same reason that I did not originally want to work on Hem-Onc—they looked terrible. Finally, they lost out yet again if their treatments failed. Our leukemia treatments worked best with young children. Nursing staff, expected to do so much for so many hurting teens, hesitated to get close to someone dying, particularly someone so much closer to their age than a child.

That was Tina's great plight. Her desperation had a reason. To this day I wonder what happened to her. When I worked Teens, I watched for her, but she never came in.

After sixteen months on Hem-Onc, caring for leukemia patients in circumstances that encouraged commitment, when I began to work with teens, the emotional distance between staff and those patients angered me. Yet I had the same problem with other illnesses. Some patients attracted my sympathy, particularly those with auto-immune diseases. Their entire lives would be dominated by problems for which they bore no responsibility. But other patients who were just as sick did not get my attention. With girls who had anorexia nervosa, I had little sympathy. I just wanted to scream at them to eat.

I wasn't alone. All the teen staff suffered from compassionate overload and compensated in different ways. With patients in so many terrible situations, we simply didn't have enough sympathy to go around. Some lost out, and that apparently included a frightened Tina. That's how we failed her. That emotional distance fed Tina's desperation. She believed those caring for her lacked the commitment she craved, hence her desperate efforts to please, efforts that made no sense.

Keep something important in mind. Tina differed from other patients in degree not kind. That is what I mean about the teaching value of intensity. Most hospitalized patients feel that they must endure situations they dislike to deserve good care. They just don't show it as obviously as Tina did. Often that means putting up with more embarrassment than is necessary.

Next, we'll look at a teen girl who came to Hem-Onc for more than a single night, and who presented a unique challenge. No other patient would shape me for the better as much as she did. Later, when I was working full-time with girls her age, I'd be thankful I had her as a patient. Amazingly gentle despite the most terrible of circumstances, she taught me much. For that I am forever grateful. Her name is Christy, and I'll never forget her.

6. GENTLE CHRISTY

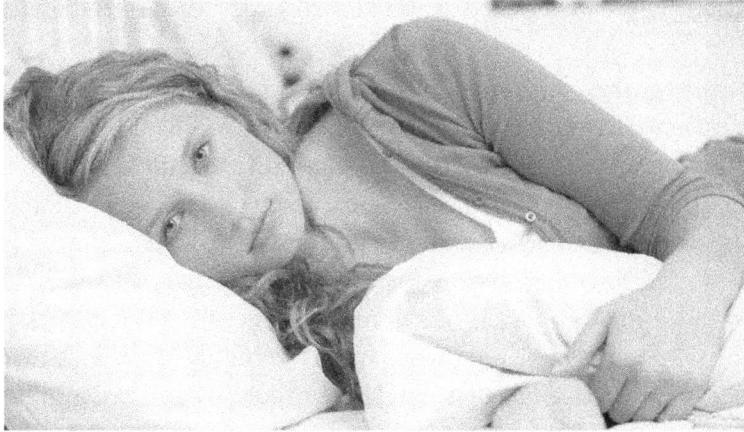

As the evening nurse described Christy's plight, I became worried. Her care would be fraught with risk. In the saddest of situations, where everything needed to go right, much could go wrong. I could blunder and hurt someone who'd had endured more than enough suffering already.

Christy was dying. Only one week shy of fifteen, she had an inoperable brain tumor. Even worse were the complications. The first was her mother, who was taking her daughter's death badly. That was why Hem-Onc, intended only for children up to nine, now had a dying teen. In her anger, the mother had treated Teens' nurses so badly, none wanted to deal with her. As the only other unit set up to care for patients in Christy's situation, we were her sole remaining hope. If we failed, her death would go even more badly.

Fortunately, the mother was not staying overnight, which suggested her grief was about herself not her daughter. Her absence made our work easier. Working nights, we were spared those angry outbursts. Given the chaos and misery when the mother was around, I resolved to do all I could to create a bubble of peace around Christy. I couldn't give her life, but I could give her a kinder death.

The second complication concerned who would care for Christy. Long before, I'd noticed a pattern. When dying children needed nurse-specific care such as morphine, the nurses were closely involved. But when a child needed only care I could provide, they stayed away, leaving everything to me. That was practical. We saw so much dying. Why get emotionally involved with a child who was about to die if it wasn't necessary? Given what I did, I never had that option. Those kids always needed me.

Brain tumors don't usually require pain medication, so Christy did not have an IV and wouldn't need a nurse. She'd be exclusively my patient. Providing her final care didn't frighten me. I knew dying children. To make no slip-ups, I saw myself as an actor taking on a role that I had to play perfectly. I liked them, focusing on their needs. I could get over the hurt of their dying. They couldn't. I responded quickly to their call light and never gave the impression I had other demands. I didn't want them to feel like a burden. I would kneel down to look eye-to-eye when I talked with them and wasn't afraid to touch them. In short, I made sure that they knew I would be with them to the end. I'd done that with little children. I could do that with Christy. Dying wasn't the issue. Something else was. Thanks to what had began with Maria, I now knew that.

The trouble lay with Christy's age and condition. The previous situations I've described—Amy, Maria, Barb, and Tina—were teen girls who had walked onto our unit and could have cared for their own needs but for a silly mindset that treated them as helplessly bedridden when they weren't. That left them and I with flexibility in embarrassing situations.

Christy was different. Her tumor meant she could do little more than roll from side to side. I'd have to help her with everything. That's why during report I thought glumly, "First, a cancer that's killing her. Then a berserk mother and eviction from a room near those her own age. Now she has her final care provided by a guy she doesn't know. Everything is going wrong for this girl."

After report, I went into Christy's room. She was gentle and soft-spoken, with light brown hair and a wonderful smile. I introduced myself and told her I'd be providing her care in the nights ahead. I also told her that, if there was anything she didn't want me to do, I'd happily get her nurse.

There was one ray of hope. Cala, with whom I shared that night Hem-Onc position, was now in her last year of nursing school.

When she'd been full-time, I wondered how she managed to work nights and attend classes the next day. Now she worked only two nights a week, so we had an arrangement. I covered weekday nights. She came in Friday and Saturday evenings, working only when she didn't have classes the next day. She'd take care of Christy the next two nights. That gave me time to think, and maybe Cala would reassure Christy about me.

That weekend, I recalled a car accident I was in a couple of years earlier. Perhaps fearing a cardiac tamponade from an impact on my chest that had sent me flying over twenty feet through the air, the paramedics rushed me to the city's premier ER, where I was quickly surrounded by staff. They wasted no time. My clothes came off at the same time IV and heart monitor cables were being placed. I recalled a nurse looking away between my clothes and gown. Even in all that confusion, I appreciated what she had done. That, I decided, was what I needed to do with Christy but with a difference. Instead of looking away, I'd look her in the eyes as much as possible. I'll explain what that means better in a later chapter.

Sunday evening, Christy became my patient again. She was so marvelously gentle and kind, I felt privileged to be with her. Some people fear caring for the dying. I often felt honored. That was particularly true with her.

If you'd had looked into Christy's room, you would have seen evidence of what she was enduring so quietly. Other teens would have rooms filled with stuffed animals, signed banners from school, bundles of flowers, and numerous foil balloons shaped like hearts. Hers was as empty as an ancient tomb. Her mother's anger had driven away friends and family. Knowing her, I could not imagine her not having a host of friends. Yet there she was, left all alone by her mother's anger, but still patient, considerate, and cooperative, even smiling when I came into her room. I never heard a word of complaint from her. In that loneliness, I became her last friend.

Christy never slept at night. From the thoughtful look on her face when I came in, I imagined she was going over her life, taking a last look back. Perhaps she also stayed awake so she could sleep while her mother was throwing fits in the day. That happened. Her mother learned nothing from being tossed off Teens. Soon there was a growing ill-will toward the mother from Hem-Onc's other shifts. Only Christy's nights remained peaceful. Until the end she remained warm and friendly. I could not have had a better patient.

Her last night came on her fifteenth birthday, much as some of us suspected it would. At report, the evening nurse informed us that Christy was in a coma, so an IV and urine catheter had been placed. My role as her sole caregiver had ended.

Going into her room just after midnight, I told myself, "She's fifteen now." She was lying on her right side, so I gently rolled her onto her left, our usual procedure to keep sores from developing. When I did that, she stopped breathing. Should I simply let her die, sparing the nurse and I an encounter with that dreadful mother? But that would leave her family out of her death and would not be right, however difficult it might be for us. So I turned her onto her back, so she could breathe more freely, added blow-by oxygen, and whispered "Breathe, Christy, breathe." Whether she heard me or not, she began to breathe again.

Her mother arrived about half an hour later. Since neither the nurse nor I had met her before, the situation did not become tense, as I'd feared. About four a.m., Christy's breathing again stopped, and her mother began to scream for us to "do something." I was glad for the nurse on duty that night. She wasn't the most technically skilled, but she had a wonderful heart. She responded marvelously, holding the mother and repeating, "Let her go. Let her go." After enduring so much, Christy was finally at peace.

Later, when a difficult situation arose, and I felt frustrated at myself for mishandling it, I would recall Christy. Thanks to her gentle personality, I got her care right. Later, something she taught me would prove vital when I faced a room filled with girls whose surgeries left them almost as helpless as she. That's coming up.

Before we take up that, however, I'll give you a quick look at what my work on Hem-Onc was like, so you'll better understand how I respond when I transferred to caring for teens full-time. I'll tell you about two special patients of mine, Jackie and Binky.

7. JACKIE AND BINKY

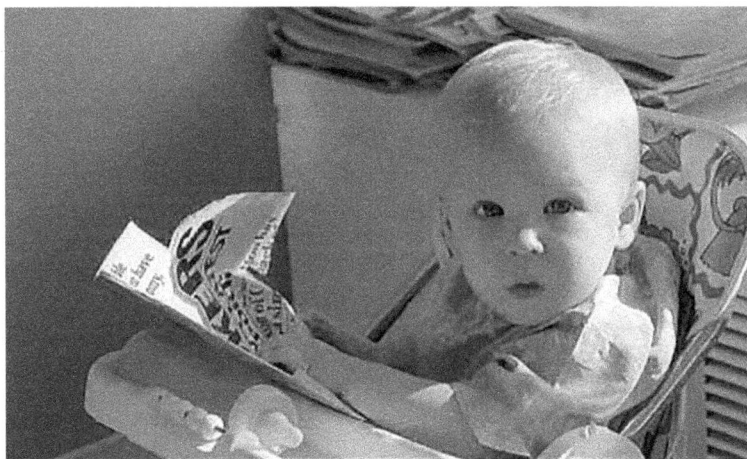

Cute isn't she. She's Jackie, my all-time favorite. I include four chapters about her in *My Nights with Leukemia*. In this book I've placed her with another favorite to correct any impression that my work was about embarrassment. It wasn't even remotely so. It was about giving life and health to adorable kids and later teens. One reason I write books such as this one is to make sure they're not forgotten. I want you to appreciate their lives.

Jackie's impossible odds began with her diagnosis. She had a leukemia so rare that at the time of her diagnosis there were only 32 cases in the medical literature. At six months, she was the youngest ever. Within hours of admission, she developed complications, with a serious infection and bleeding from her just-installed central line. She was transferred to the ICU, where she was given a less than two percent chance of leaving alive. An ICU nurse told me that only Jackie's obvious determination to live kept them treating her. They could not give up, because she refused to give up.

Jackie cared nothing for such odds. After six weeks in our ICU, she'd recovered enough to return to Hem-Onc, although her troubles were far from over. Wondering about an anti-viral drug she was receiving, I looked it up. The description opened with the FDA's well-known black box warning. Bold text in a thick black box made clear this drug was only to be given in life-threatening emergencies. The long-term complications were so terrible, it was used only when a patient would die without it. That's how serious her infection was. Jackie's other trouble was her cancer. It's rareness and her young age meant our specialists had no idea how to treat it. With no better alternative, they gave her our standard leukemia treatment. It would be a shot in the dark.

That's when I came in. "Of all the kids you've cared for," I asked myself, "why fall the hardest for the one with the poorest prognosis?" Sensing that, one nurse asked what I'd do if Jackie died. I didn't know, I told her. For our other children, their death was like entering a dark tunnel, knowing I'd return into the light. With Jackie, I could see only darkness stretching far ahead. When she asked why Jackie was special, I replied, "Because we're both stubborn." Yes, like attracts like. One stubborn person was coming to the aid of another. Together, we would lick that awful leukemia.

Fortunately, there was much I could do for little Miss Stubborn. I resolved to give her every moment I could spare. Nothing escaped my attention. If she as much as burped, I asked why. Her struggle in the ICU hadn't left much time for nutrition. She came to us so weak that at nine months she couldn't hold a bottle. I resolved to hold it for her, so she could catch up. As you can see from the picture at the start of this chapter, six weeks later she was much stronger.

I grabbed that feeding time whenever I could. One night it came just after 4 a.m., when the nurse had left on break. I'd just settled down with Jackie and her bottle, when another child's IV pump beeped. I left to take care of that, and when I returned, Jackie was a little miffed. Then another IV beeped. Starting to get upset myself, I again fixed the problem and returned to an obviously angry little baby. The third time it'd happened, I realized what was going on. Before the nurse left, she had ran all her 4 a.m. medications and started the follow-up rinses. Flipping the IVs back to maintenance was left to me. Before I returned to Jackie, I checked every IV on Hem-Onc, making sure there would be no more beeps. By that point, Jackie was so ticked off at me for having abandoned her three times, that for the rest of that night she refused to look at me. "That's OK," I told her, "you know I like you."

After feeding I'd rock her to sleep, so she got as much rest as possible. Being lullaby-challenged, I only knew the chorus to one song, which I sang over and over in my terrible voice, one only babies appreciate. Although I didn't realize it at the time, the last line was especially appropriate.

You are my sunshine, my only sunshine.
You make me happy when skies are grey.
You'll never know dear, how much I love you.
Please don't take my sunshine away.

To my great delight, my sunshine wasn't taken away. She fought off that viral infection and went through chemotherapy better than most. The picture you see was taken about six weeks after she'd returned to Hem-Onc. She's healthy and strong. Knowing she'd soon be discharged, one morning just before day shift arrived, we held a going-away party. She got to tear pages out of old magazines, while I took pictures of a most brave little baby.

After I'd transferred to Teens, Jackie's mother brought her to see me. The instant she saw her nighttime buddy, she leapt out of her mother's arms and into mine. Even better news followed. She never relapsed. Later, she would reach a critical milestone—five years leukemia-free. Today she runs several small businesses, which I'm sure she does with her usual determination. Nothing stops her.

Jackie wasn't my only special patient. Binky was another favorite—and that of every nurse who cared for him. I still remember the first time he and I met. As I came up to his bed, I saw a homemade sign at the foot saying, "I know I'm special because God don't make no junk." I would soon learn how true that was.

Binky looked much like the Kermit the Frog doll that often lay on his bed. With an enlarged belly and thin, spindly arms and legs, he had prune belly syndrome, accompanied by only one barely functioning kidney. With no working bladder, his urine dripped out, one drop at a time from an opening on his stomach. He wasn't always that weak. I saw pictures of him from a time when he was strong enough to stand on his own. But by the time I knew him, he'd deteriorated to the point where he had to be propped up with pillows.

Binky was loved by everyone who cared for him, and the reason was obvious. One day, an order came to pull his NG tube. I was doing that as painlessly as possibly, planning to pull slowly until the tip reached his throat and then move quickly through the gag zone. That took great care. Sensing my concern, he stopped me and said that I shouldn't feel bad about what I had to do, that he was OK. That concern for his caregivers is what endeared him to nurses. Nurses like being appreciated. He melted their hearts.

With but one failing kidney, Binky came in often. He was one of a small group of dying children whose behavior mystified me. Despite going through terrible suffering, these amazing children would thank me for each little thing I did. At first, I felt like saying, "Oh, it's nothing. They pay me to do this." Why this exceptional thoughtfulness?, I wondered. If they'd been angry or irritable, I would have understood.

Then it came to me what was happening. Imagine that you're five years old and know you'll soon die. All that you will accomplish in the rest of your life will take place in the next few weeks with the few who come to your bedside. Their kindness to us was an attempt to give meaning to their tragically shortened lives. That's why it mattered that we graciously accept their thanks. That's also why I write about them. They should not be forgotten.

After Binky died, his family held a memorial service for staff. They choose the best possible time, which was early afternoon. But that was best only because it inconvenienced all shifts equally. Those on nights had to get up at what was to us about 3 a.m. Those on days had to find someone to come early and cover for them. Those on evenings had to find someone to stay over until they could arrive late. Everyone had to make a substantial sacrifice to attend.

For Hem-Onc children, typically four to six nursing staff would attend a funeral. How many attended Binky's memorial service? I didn't need to count, because a nurse did it for me. Twenty-four members of the hospital's staff went to great effort to honor Binky's short but meaningful life. He was every bit as special as that sign had said. With him, God had not made junk.

Now we'll move with me to Teens, with its often grouchy boys, to see what they can teach us.

8. GROUCHY BOYS

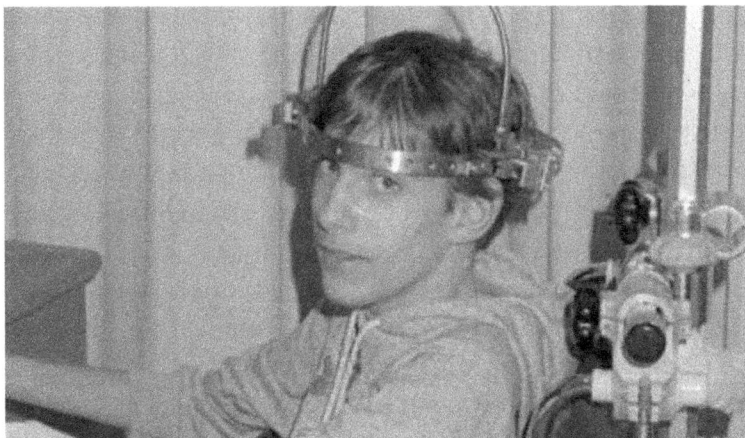

Just after I transferred to Teens, I noticed a hint that the complications of working with teenagers, although rarely discussed, were well understood. Someone had put a cheap plastic 3-D painting in our snack room. I featured a little boy and girl facing away, so their bare bottoms stood out in the plastic, but with their faces also turned toward the artist. Tacky but true. Exposure like that is a part the work at any hospital, but these almost-adult teens added to the complications and sometimes the humor.

When I first arrived in late spring, embarrassment was the least of my worries. Going from nights on Hem-Onc to days on Teens meant new stresses that hit me far harder than embarrassment. On Hem-Onc I finished up a seven-day stretch on a Sunday morning and entered a new seven-day stretch on Teens the next morning. That meant working fourteen days without a break and, since those days were split between two pay periods, I received no overtime pay.

On Hem-Onc, almost all my patients were children with leukemia. That's an extremely serious illness, but only one illness with standard treatments. In contrast, on Teens my patients had every illness imaginable and, as I mentioned earlier, often the worst cases of such illnesses. That complexity and severity meant added stress. Without the benefit of a new orientation, I now faced caring for serious illnesses I knew little about. That I did not like.

My status also changed. When Cala graduated from nursing school and left, I became the most senior staff on Hem-Onc, with more experience than *all* the night-shift nurses and residents *combined*. I'd worked Hem-Onc almost exclusively for sixteen months, while nurses and residents passed through. When decisions were made, what I said carried weight. Not so on Teens, where I was the newest staff member and would remain so for my entire ten months. I had responsibility but little authority. That meant more stress.

There was also a different work culture. On nights, hospital politics mattered little. What happened on nights, stayed on nights. What happened on days, I soon discovered, often got someone hot and bothered. Nights was a party among a select few. Days was a giant minefield, bringing still more stress.

Nights on Hem-Onc resembled how like soldiers describe war—long hours of dull routine broken by seconds of sheer terror. Round and round I went, checking on my seven little cuties. New orders, admissions and discharges were rare. When something happened, it was serious. The heart of my job was staying alert through seemingly endless nights to catch the early signs of a crisis. Even a brief delay might make the difference between life and death.

In contrast, days on Teens were an unending struggle. It was chaotic, with orders changing and patients coming and going. Our teens had every imaginable illness. Most important of all, my patients had changed. On Hem-Onc, all were children. Frightened by an illness beyond their understanding, they were scared, so I focused on winning their trust. Once that was established, all went well. That was one reason I loved the work.

On Teens, I soon realized I didn't have one patient population. I had three to contend with. The first were kids from ten to puberty. They were much like the older children I'd cared for on Hem-Onc, so I understood them well. There were a few modesty issues, including a difficult one I describe soon, but not many.

At puberty, as many parents know, that world flipped upside down. My patients were not only different, the gap between boys and girls grew enormous. Walking between a multi-bed room with four teen boys to one with four girls was like traveling between two radically different countries. To someone used to the much smaller differences between little boys and girls, that was confusing.

Our teen boys were like the citizens of a grim Northern European country where the sun never shines. Smiles were rare and conversations were brief. The only exceptions were boys with long-term problems. You see the picture of one such boy at the start of this chapter, halo traction and all. Bill's back was in such bad shape, he was told that his surgery had a fifty/fifty chance of leaving him paralyzed. With impressive guts, he went ahead and the result was a spectacular success. He was great to talk with. Unfortunately, most teen guys weren't open. Many were withdrawn and grouchy.

His friendliness hints at the root of the problem. Boys with lengthy illnesses were over feeling powerless. Our other teen boys, most in a hospital for the first time, hated their dependence. They were becoming men. They wanted to be respected as men not mothered like sick little boys. Not getting that, they sulked and pouted.

Even worse, we did not make their adjustment easy. Staffing was one reason. One of my first thoughts after starting Teens was, "Wow, so many pretty nurses!" Without exception, every nurse was attractive. Later, I'd realize there was a practical reason for that. The work was so demanding, only young and athletic nurses could keep up. That almost guaranteed they'd be pretty.

Now imagine you're a sixteen-year-old boy surrounded by nurses who look like cheerleaders. You'd want to impress them, wouldn't you? Ah, but look at your pitiful state. Not very impressive. Heck, you can't even pee without asking for a urinal. Then there were all the orthopedic surgeries we did with their aftermath of dependency. As a boy, you might be stuck in bed, as helpless as a newborn baby. That was one reason for their unhappiness—all those pretty nurses they couldn't impress. Feel sorry for them. I sometimes did.

There is nothing unique about the response of those boys. After I had written a draft of this chapter, I read Erich Remarque's description of what it was like to be a German soldier in World War I in his bestselling *All Quiet on the Western Front* (German: 1928, English: 1929). In the tenth chapter, his central character is wounded and placed on a hospital train, where he is cared for by nurses who're called "sisters." Notice what happens.

At night I cannot sleep. Kropp is restless too. The train rides easily over the rails. I cannot realize it all yet; a bed, a train, home. "Albert!" I whisper.

"Yes…"

"Do you know where the latrine is?"

"Over to the right of the door, I think."

"I'm going to have a look." It is dark, I grope for the edge of the bed and cautiously try to slide down. But my foot finds no support, I begin to slip, the plaster leg is no help, and with a crash I lie on the floor.

"Damn!" I say.

"Have you bumped yourself?" asks Kropp.

"You could hear that well enough for yourself," I growl, "my head…."

A door opens in the rear of the car. The sister comes with a light and looks at me.

"He has fallen out of bed…"

She feels my pulse and smooths my forehead. "You haven't a fever, though."

"No," I agree.

"Have you been dreaming then?" she asks.

"Perhaps…" I evade. The interrogation starts again. She looks at me with her clear eyes, and the more wonderful and sweet she is the less am I able to tell her what I want.

I am lifted up into bed again. That will be all right. As soon as she goes, I must try to climb down again. If she were an old woman, it might be easier to say what a man wants, but she is so very young, at the most twenty-five, it can't be done. I can't possibly tell her.

Then Albert comes to my rescue, he is not bashful, it makes no difference to him who is upset. He calls to the sister. She turns round. "Sister, he wants…" but no more does Albert know how to express it modestly and decently. Out there we say it in a single word, but here, to such a lady… All at once he remembers his school days and finishes hastily: "He wants to leave the room, sister."

"Ah!" says the sister, "but he shouldn't climb out of his bed with his plaster bandage. What do you want then?" she says, turning to me.

I am in mortal terror at this new turn, for I haven't any idea what the things are called professionally. She comes to my help.

"Little or big?"

This shocking business! I sweat like a pig and say shyly: "Well, only quite a little one…"

At any rate, it produces the effect.

I get a bottle. After a few hours I am no longer the only one, and by morning we are quite accustomed to it and ask for what we want without any false modesty.

Notice that those battle-hardened soldiers had the same problem as our teen boys, but take note that theirs was faced and resolved. Sadly, ours never was. Hospitals should end this false modesty.

My fellow assistants created a different problem. All but me were middle-aged women returning to work after raising children. They were the age of these boys' mothers, creating yet more emotional conflicts. Think of a boy's terrible plight. When he needed a urinal, he had to ask either a cheerleader or a mother. That may be why, when I entered a boys' room, often three of the four would ask for their urinal. Being a guy helped, but far less than I thought.

That urinal problem suggests one answer. Instead of putting it out of sight and making patients ask for it, why not place it where a patient can get it for himself? It could be horizontal when empty. Once used, it could be turned up, so staff know to empty it. There's no reason hospitals can't make voiding less embarrassing.

Here we must not pretend the two sexes are identical. These boys wanted to respond to stress with an aggressive fight or flight. Unfortunately, that only made their plight worse. Who were they going to punch in the nose? No one, certainly not those pretty nurses or kind mothers. How could they run away when confined to a bed and often in traction? They couldn't. Unable to use wired-in macho responses, most fled into a shell, emotionally and socially. They talked as little as possible and barely cooperated, even with me. Often, I could only get them to follow orders by nagging.

Another factor hearkened back to boyhood frustrations. Imagine a boy of four who wants play in street with his toy truck, but his mother, being the sensible sort, won't let him. If she were mean, rebelling would be easy. But he knows she loves him, and that makes the rules he wants to break all the more galling. Hospitalized as teens, that long-ago frustration resurfaces. Kindness only made the restrictions we imposed worse. Our teen boys felt like little boys again, and our staff became like their long-ago mothers, hence their unspoken rebellion. That's why older men aren't likely to respond quite the same. Someone who is the father of three and the owner of a business with two-hundred employees doesn't worry about being mistaken for a boy. He may, however, resent being ordered about, rather than giving orders.

Embarrassment made the powerlessness of these teen boys even more obvious. They were surrounded by women, so much so that they rebelled against these all-seeing females. Except for a few who were unconscious, they resembled a city under siege. I was both amused and saddened by the result. All wore their underpants without exception. All kept their gowns tucked in. Even on the hottest days, all kept their sheets pulled up. They were miserable and, since I wasn't the cause, I couldn't do a thing about it.

Some nurses made matters worse, although it isn't fair to blame them. They had little choice. Imagine Sally the Nurse. She's a cute five-foot-two and weighs but a hundred-and-ten pounds. Her orders say she must do something to Sam the Giant, a six-foot-four high-school quarterback who weights twice as much as she. What's a nurse to do, particularly given that the guy is likely to be uncooperative? She rushes in and pounces, doing what she must before he can resist. No wonder these guys seemed paranoid. In their circumstances, I'd feel the same. Feel sorry for the nurses too. They had a tough job. They did not want to do what they often had to do.

When I first started, I thought embarrassment issues would come down hard on me. Anytime a guy needed to poop, I'd be called in to assist, even if he wasn't my patient. To my surprise, that never happened. These put-upon guys felt too powerless to make demands. That added to their misery.

Soon after I started, I began to feel sorry for both sexes—the guys because I could do so little about their plight and the girls because my male presence was their plight. The best illustration of the differences came with a common problem—the need some patients had to get to the toilet with our assistance. Often, there would be a surgeon's order that they must get up on a certain day, like it or not, to qualify for discharge.

For some, both boys and girls, the first time they stood up after surgery was extremely painful. I knew how they felt. A couple of years before I had been in an auto accident that pulled almost every muscle from my waist up. For about a week afterward, getting up in the morning was sheer misery. When I sat up in bed, I'd spend about a minute gasping for breath. Standing meant another minute of terrible pain. Since I was at home, I had to get myself to the toilet. Worried about falls, the hospital permitted no such independence. For those patients, we kept their side rails up, so we controlled when they got up. They had to go through us and only with our help.

Some boys were so large, I wondered how I'd stop their fall. I decided that I had to correct their balance in the first split-second, or both they and I were going down onto the hard linoleum. No girl raised that issue. Some were so light, I could have carried them to the toilet much like we did children on the medical unit, perching the littlest ones high up on a child's toilet designed for kids seven and up. And no, I didn't do that with those girls.

Teen boys and girls responded differently. The boys did their best to conceal their pain. It was a rare opportunity to show their macho, and they made the most of it. With them, I said nothing as we walked, since they'd take that as insulting. No guy ever wanted my assistance sitting down. That was too demeaning. Fortunately, there was no reason for me to insist. If they were willing to endure the pain, they could take care of themselves.

The girls were different. They were happy for my assistance and weren't ashamed to grimace as we walked ever so slowly toward the toilet. With them, I kept up a steady chatter of small talk to get their mind off the pain. What I said mattered so little, I can't even remember the topics. If I were in the same situation today, I might play a game called, "What's your favorite?" I'd go first, asking her a question like, "What's your favorite pizza?" After she answered, it would be her turn to ask me a favorite. That would offer the distraction she needed.

What came next needs an explanation. Our toilet-only rooms were designed for safety above all else. They were small, barely larger than the toilet itself. That was clever, because it made falling almost impossible. On every side were sturdy chrome handrails. The toilets were even wheelchair accessible, since the wide door made it possible to slide sideways from outside onto the toilet seat. But there was a serious hitch. The tight space meant there was no way to help those girls onto a toilet without embarrassment. I could not stand in front of them and slip down their undies beneath their gown like I did when they were in bed. Assistance had to come from behind.

Compared to the dull uniformity of male macho, these girls were more flexible. On one hand, I was a guy, so helping them sit meant exposure. On the other hand, by quickly easing them onto that seat, I reduced their pain to just a split-second. It's a classic illustration of what I tell readers in *Hospital Gowns*. Being hospitalized, I wrote, often means choosing between pain and embarrassment. You must choose. I stress that as patients they should to make clear which they want. If they want help, they should say so. If they don't, they should explain that they can handle the sitting themselves.

Since these girls hadn't read my as-yet unwritten book, neither they nor I found talking about the situation easy. Instead, I gave them a couple of seconds to decide. Those who stood waiting for my help got it and didn't appear to mind. For those who moved inside and seemed intent on seating themselves, I closed the door. That worked well enough.

Walking the occasional post-op boy or girl to the toilet became one of my first learning experiences on Teens. The guys were so difficult and stubborn, I will attempt to make sense of them in the next chapter. The girls were easier than I expected, although I would soon discover that when a girl became complicated, she became very complicated. I still had a lot to learn. You will find out about that in the chapter about Min. But first we need to take a closer look at male attitudes, particularly in the face of danger or under the stress of hospitalization.

9. Bonding Brothers

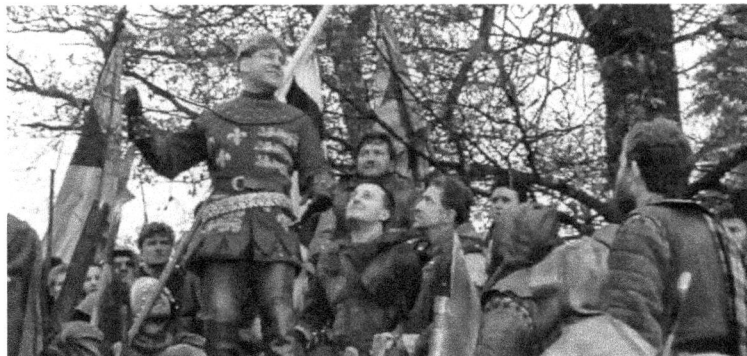

Taking a break from writing a few years ago, I was walking around Seattle's Green Lake, when I saw something that troubled me so badly, I turned around and walked past it again. No, this isn't my imagination, I thought. I saw fear in the eyes of mothers pushing strollers.

What frightened those young mothers was a guy clumsily throwing knives at a tree only a few yards from a walkway filled with people. Like those mothers, I had no trouble imagining a knife bouncing off the tree and into the eye of a child.

The waterfront activity center was nearby. Surely, I thought, the city must have a policy about such things. It did. The staff told me they'd been ordered to do nothing in such situations, not even to call the police. No doubt the city's lawyers feared a lawsuit. If you wonder why I'm no fan of lawyers, that's one reason.

I walked back toward Mr. Jerk. I couldn't expect a mother with little children to confront a man armed with knives and twice her weight, so that left me. In the past, I had worked with addicts, alcoholics, and the mentally ill. I knew how to handle touchy situations. Maybe I could persuade Mr. Jerk to pick a different tree. On the way, I asked man to watch and call the police if trouble developed. Without a word, Mr. Chicken darted away. "Worthless," I thought.

As calmly as I could, I suggested to Mr. Jerk that he find a different tree. When he refused, I warned him I'd call the police. When he behaved oddly, I backed away while calling 911. Only then did I realized that he had four inches in height and about forty pounds on me, not to mention those knifes. Fortunately, as he began to move toward me, Mr. Big, far taller than Mr. Jerk, intercepted him and made clear I wasn't to be bothered.

Shortly afterward, Mr. Big and I talked, each eager to show our appreciation. He'd seen what I'd seen, but hesitated to act until I did. I was just as appreciative, thanking him for preventing what could have been a dangerous confrontation. We formed a mutual admiration society sometimes called male bonding.

Notice that male bonding isn't just men doing something together, say fishing or playing cards. It's what results when they face a shared danger and each learns he can depend on the other. In *Henry V*, Shakespeare explains what that means in his famous St. Crispin's Day speech, delivered by the English king just before his exhausted men must face a French army five times their size.

We few, we happy few, we band of brothers;
For he to-day that sheds his blood with me
Shall be my brother; be he ne'er so vile,
This day shall gentle his condition:
And gentlemen in England now a-bed
Shall think themselves accursed they were not here,
And hold their manhoods cheap whiles any speaks
That fought with us upon Saint Crispin's day.

Understand that, and you'll grasp the frustrations of our teen boys when their surgery left them stranded in bed unable to show their manhood, much like those unfortunate "gentlemen in England now a-bed." We expected to them lie there, while we did everything for them, even what they found humiliating. That's why they sulked, much like those "accursed" men who had not "fought with us upon Saint Crispin's day." They resented being treated as helpless little boys. Mr. Big and I felt great after vanquishing Mr. Jerk. Our teen boys had no reason to feel manly.

Imagine a medieval joust with our boys as participants. That was like the sports and showing off on motorcycles that had led to their surgery. Their longing to impress girls at their high school was no different from the desire knights at a joust had to impress lovely maidens. Yet look at where their "jousting" had gotten them. They were often strung up in traction, forced to ask for a urinal, and fretting that their undies might show. That's not masculine and is why our boys were so unhappy. We weren't offering them a role they wanted to play. They had to engage in the most unheroic activity imaginable—lying in bed like a sick little boy dependent on his mommy to go pee-pee. Yes, that bad. While these teen boys needed praise for cooperating, it should *never* be for going pee-pee.

Despite my fumbling efforts, those boys remained distant and uncommunicative. Getting them to obey even the smallest of orders often took nagging. Why, I thought, are they being like this? I can understand why embarrassment might lead them to be reticent around our women staff. But why all that unhappiness?

To understand, first recall the delight Mr. Big and I felt to discover, when we faced that knife-tossing Mr. Jerk, that we could depend on one another. That's because male bonding isn't universal. Bonding to some males is folly. They can't be depended on, much like Mr. Chicken. Shakespeare has Henry V express a similar feeling toward men unwilling to face the coming battle.

Rather proclaim it, Westmoreland, through my host,
That he which hath no stomach to this fight,
Let him depart; his passport shall be made
And crowns for convoy put into his purse:
We would not die in that man's company
That fears his fellowship to die with us.

Shakespeare put it perfectly. A bond between men requires a test of courage. Pass that test, and the bond is made. That's Mr. Big and I. When there is a failure to display courage, rejection soon follows. That's the clucking Mr. Chicken.

In our more decadent age, it's easy to forget just how necessary that is. When a man ventured out on rough seas in a small boat to feed his family, he needed to know that those with him would not panic in a storm. When he hunted a dangerous beast or faced battle, he needed to know that those he was with would stand by him. Male bonding places men side by side, facing a common foe. Each may bring different talents to the fight, but as Shakespeare's Henry V put it, shared danger makes them brothers. That's wired into the right sort of men. And yes, some males—I don't call them men—don't have that wiring. Many of them are evil, preying on the weak, much as we will see in later with the plight of young women traveling in Europe.

Major surgery is as much a test of strength as facing battle, so we should look at the fight those hospitalized boys faced. We expected them to face the pain and boredom alone, without bonding to other men and indeed without a challenge that demanded brave deeds from them. That left them feeling useless, and the situation wasn't helped by our female staff, whose forced-upon-them bonding was that of a mommy for a little boy. That's why they were unhappy. That's why they felt humiliated. That is why they withdrew. Their embarrassment was acute, extending far beyond mere exposure.

Could something be done for them? I've asked myself that question many times. One answer only applies to a particular set of circumstances, but it suggests other possibilities. These boys needed a hospital-based challenge they could face and emerge victorious. Here's an example.

Hem-Onc was seven beds in a larger medical unit. I wasn't the only one to sense the need for a specialized pediatric cancer unit. Later, the hospital would dedicate that entire unit to cancer, mixing teens with children. I asked myself what I'd have done if I'd been a sixteen-year-old boy with leukemia. I could, of course, withdraw and obsess over my helplessness and misfortune, much like those boys who'd had major surgeries did. That I would find disgusting. Were I such a boy, I told myself, I'd refuse to fret about whether I'd live or die. God and the treatment itself would decide that. I'd befriend the smaller children and do what I could to encourage them. I'd refuse to focus on myself and live in a too-small world.

That's where our problem lay. Our teen boys were offered no alternative but to obsess over themselves. That's why they were miserable. Hospitals should find ways to help them escape that morass and become useful and constructive, even when trapped in bed. They want to do something that matters. Give them that chance. That'll take creativity, but it can be done.

Later, we'll take a similarly broad look at our girls. But for now, we will look at a particular girl's experience, one that, as difficult as it was, would teach me much.

10. Modest Min

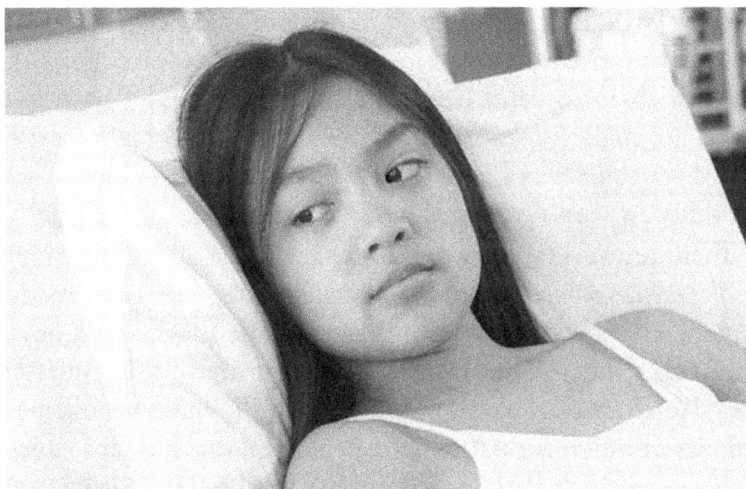

Min was Asian and tiny even for eleven. I gave her that name because it's one Chinese parents give a daughter who's quick and sensitive. Min's back surgery had been so serious, she was wearing a body cast from just above her knees up to her neck and almost out to her elbows. She was completely helpless, which was why her lovely eyes filled with fear when I came to her bed.

I was afraid too. To prevent sores, she needed to be rotated every two hours. To flip her over, I would slide her to the far side of the bed and then roll her inside that body cast like a mummy. One slip, I worried, and she might tumble back and flop off the bed, doing terrible harm to her fragile back and perhaps leaving her paralyzed for life. Working in a hospital, being paranoid helps.

Min feared something else. She was aware that her cast had two openings in the usual places. I knew that too because for two hours each day a surgical nurse took her out of that cast, so it could dry out. That's when I saw it uncovered. I did what I could to ease her fears, but I faced a major problem. Other staff, meaning women, almost certainly yanked away the sheet that was her only covering when they turned her. That saved time and trouble. I didn't, but continually adjusting that sheet while flipping was fraught with risk. What could I have done?

Her mother might have helped. But she was also tiny and seemed to know little English. Asking her might make matters worse and could have caused the very embarrassment Min feared. I could have talked to Min to calm her fears. But what could I have said that would not make her more afraid? Not knowing what to say, I muddled through as best I could. Poor girl, stuck with clueless, new-to-teens me. At least nothing she feared happened.

There are several answers to the fears of patients we might call the *frightened modest*. One, I will save for later, one I've already mentioned ('what's your favorite' game), and one I'll mention now, since its impetus must come from a level well above floor nursing. For everyone from doctors to the nursing staff, there should be a formal classification for patients such as Min, one perhaps called VSP for Very Sensitive Patient. It wouldn't need to be widely advertised, but would simplify decisions. For Min, it'd mean flips were always done by same-sex staff behind drawn curtains. It'd also be useful for patients who've suffered sexual abuse and fear losing control. Both situations should matter enough for hospitals to adopt the proper formal policies and encourage staff to follow them.

Min was a early revelation of what working on Teens was going to be like. Thanks to her, I realized that these girls, who were half my work, could prove complicated. Recall my limited experience up to that point, and how contradictory it had been. The few teen girls I'd had as patients could hardly have been more different. They ranged from Min, terrified of any exposure, to an angry Barb, with her "no way," and on to Tina, whose desperation overwhelmed her modesty, as well as shy Maria and gentle Christy. How was I to know mere seconds after our first meeting which kind of girl I was dealing with? I couldn't. Was I fated to blunder from patient to patient, never getting it right? I hated that. I liked these girls.

Fortunately, what I did right built on what I had learned with the kids on Hem-Onc. That was the importance of being reassuring and building trust. That made as much difference with embarrassment as it did with pain. Here's one illustration.

Imagine that you're a girl named Traci. You are fifteen and just had an appendectomy. The hospital dictates the outer clothes you wear—that dreadful gown—so undies are the only way to express your individuality. To celebrate, you're wearing your favorite panties, tiny and decorated with cute dancing bunnies. You've just woken up on the morning after your surgery when a guy dressed like nursing staff comes into the room. That's me, almost as new to Teens as you.

"Oh, my gosh," you think. "The nurse the evening before flipped my gown all the way up to check my surgery, showing everything. Will he do the same? If he does, I'll just die." Yes, very teen girlish.

You watch him carefully as he moves about the room. None of the other girls panic, and they were here before you. None has their gowns flung over their heads, but then they've not just has surgeries. Finally, he comes up to you. "What will he do?," you wonder.

Traci's situation was one of my first when I began working with teens. Once or twice a week, a girl would be recovering from a surgery, which, if she needed to stay overnight, was typically abdominal. I'd taken care of only a few surgical patients on the medical unit, but along the way I'd picked up a rule that such patients should be checked for at least two days after their surgery, looking for bleeding or for a redness that might mean infection. Some nurses did that themselves, but most depended on me. Since I didn't know which was which, I checked surgical sites with vital signs.

I'd seen how some nurses did checks. With boys, they would rush up, giving little chance to resist their quick, under-the-gown peek. That was excusable. After all, these nurses were dealing with uncooperative boys. With girls, our nurses often overdid the exposure, giving every appearance of assuming the surgeon had tried incisions in several places about a girl's tummy before recalling that an appendix was in the lower-right quadrant. One nurse told me she did that because she wanted to "see everything."

That's why this fictional Traci had reason to worry when I came into her room. Would I toss most of her gown aside to see everything? Girl-nurse with girl-patient, that might be OK. But I suspected these girls did not want me seeing much, especially those dancing bunnies. What was I to do? I didn't want them cowering under their sheets like our boys. That would leave me with almost no one to talk with. Remember, I hated day's endless busy work. The nurse and I had little time to talk. Getting to know patients was my only joy, and in practice that meant mostly these girls.

What I did with these teen girls was like what I'd done with a new child on Hem-Onc. I gave them time to adjust to me. With the kids, I often checked their IV pump first. In a multi-bed girl's room, I would save the new surgery girl for last. When I eventually came to her, I didn't rush. Sometimes embarrassment is lessened by being done as quickly as possible. Seating on a toilet is like that. That first surgery check was a situation where moving slowly and chattering about trivia worked best. Rushing in would make the girl feel the situation was spiraling beyond her control. Moving slowly gave her time to say no, although none did.

With Traci, vital signs came first. On little kids, the pulse at their wrist was hard to feel, so we counted it and respirations by plopping a stethoscope on their chests. That's fine with a child. From the first teen girl I cared for on, I knew that was not a good idea. I took an older girl's pulse with a 15-second count at her wrist. Then I took another 15 seconds, still holding her wrist, to count her respirations out of the corner of my eyes. No staring allowed.

Having done vital signs, it was time to check Traci's surgical site, which was often low on her tummy. Rather than yanking down her sheets and tossing up her gown to be done quickly, I first checked a small bag that typically hung beneath her bed and was used to drain off fluids. That done, I followed its line up, pealing back just enough gown from the side to see what I must see. No dancing bunnies, just that suture site. For all their faults, one of the advantages of hospital gowns is that they allow selective uncovering. That started Traci's day off right and established trust. My initial hour or two on the first day of caring for these girls was critical.

As odd as it sounds, girls at the extremes were the easiest. Even though she shouldn't, Tina in her desperation, would do anything. I had to draw the lines. Barb was also easy. She would refuse almost anything, making my work simple. I certainly wasn't going to rip that blanket out of her arms just to take her weight. Even Min, with her extreme modesty, was easy in one sense. She was so obviously frightened, I knew to be careful. Looking back, I should have asked the nurse I was working with to do Min's flips.

Min was among the *frightened modest*. She was dreadfully afraid of exposure and yet lacked the resolve to protect herself. Did I have other girls like her? None were as helpless as she was in that body cast. But it seems unlikely someone as modest as she would appear in my first month, but not in the nine that followed. Yet I can't recall a single situation where a girl seemed afraid. Why was that?

That's because there's a second category that might be called the *determined modest*. My failure with Min bothered me so much, I took great care thereafter. Some girls were naturally strong-willed enough not to be pushed around—grumpy Barb with her "no way" being one example. Others were clever enough to manage situations. They're the sensible girls I mention in the chapters that follow. I lowered the determination threshold enough that even the shyest felt in control, and I used ideas from the sensible to help the others.

As a result, we got along marvelously. The modest relaxed because they knew I wouldn't push. I relaxed because I knew their modesty was about themselves rather than me. None were afraid, which was a great relief. I even saw hints they were happier with a man who was careful rather than a woman who might be careless.

There is another group we might call the *learned modest*. They began like most patients, enduring exposures they dislike. But unlike most, they had health issues that meant repeated hospital visits. That led to a split between boys and girls.

Since almost all our nursing staff were female, boys had nowhere to turn when their privacy was threatened, leading to that siege mentality. Most never got beyond that. But a few faced hospitalization often enough that they concluded exposure was no big deal. They lightened up enough to be friendly.

Girls faced similar issues, but the preponderance of female caregivers had the opposite effect. Put yourself into the mind of a teen girl whose medical condition means she's hospitalized every few months. When she comes in, men on staff see her ill-clad. That's hospital care. She has nothing against them, and none strike her as creepy. The procedures are ones she's gone through more times than she can count. But that's the very point. "Other girls my age aren't having to deal with these repeated embarrassments," she tells herself, "so why should I?" Then this girl realizes something. Women are common enough, all she need do is ask that the embarrassing stuff be done by them. In a hospital you often get what you insist on, so that demand is easily accomplished. Also, since there were only a handful of these girls over those ten months, their nurses weren't overworked. They helped with their care too, often dressing and doing other tasks for themselves. That lessened the burden.

At this point I must explain something. I liked caring for these more modest girls. Their clear boundaries made my job easier. The fact that girls so sensitive to intrusions relaxed assured me that none saw me as a creep. In those early weeks before I developed confidence, that mattered.

But I also liked the casual girls that we're about to take up. I may give the chapters about them titles such as "Dratted Bedpans" and "Hated Linens," but my frustrations were directed at procedures not patients. I also can't praise them enough. I was flattered by their trust. Over time I learned to enjoy the challenges of caring for them. They taught me much.

Finally, keep in mind that distinctions between casual and modest weren't rigid. Even the most casual had their limits, as "Hated Linens" illustrates. At the opposite extreme, when they felt secure, even the most modest could accept a gown change and respond with one of those "Beautiful Smiles."

Now prepare for a dramatic transition. Bored and tired, the next girls we discuss are not modest. They kick down their sheets and roll about in an effort to find comfort in their miserably hot room. They and I will face a host of issues together.

11. FLOPPING GOWNS

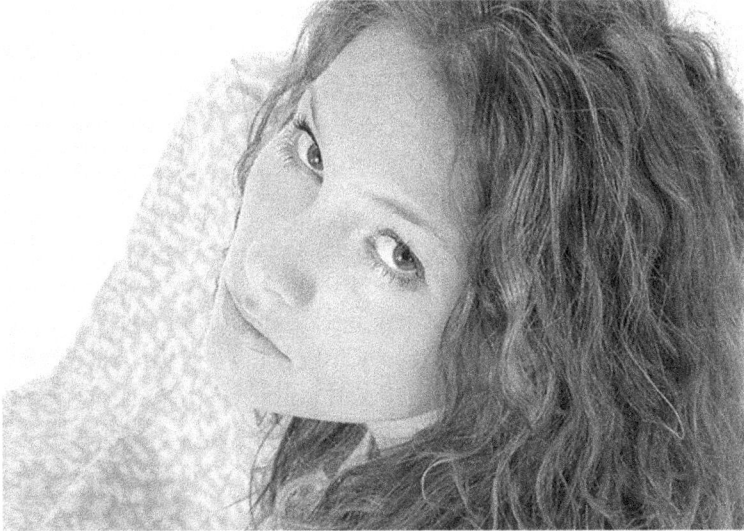

Throughout that May, my first month with teens, the nursing staff discussed what was coming. Summer was our busy season. Orthopedic surgery, common in teens, was one of our specialties. Whenever possible, the most demanding of those surgeries were scheduled over the summer when our patients were out of school. The most serious were scheduled first, so those patients would have the most time to recover. That's why Min came before school was out. Having worked primarily with kids who had leukemia, I knew little about surgery. Come June, I would get my baptism of fire.

Most boys facing major surgeries were placed in a four-bed room on C cluster. Their surgeries were typically to correct either sports injuries or stupid things done on motorcycles. Many required traction, which made their care still more awkward. Despite the heat, they kept themselves well-covered. Modesty trumped comfort.

Many of the girls' surgeries were for scoliosis, an excessive curvature of the spine. Some cases can be treated with braces and exercise. Others require spinal fusion, a surgery so complex it can last six to eight hours. At that time, their back was opened up from their shoulder blades to their hips, and their spine straightened by any means necessary. Online, you can find amazing before and after x-rays. Notice the extreme curves in their spines before, and afterward all the metal hardware these girls will carry for the rest of their lives. Often that meant two long stainless steel rods running down their backbone with a couple of dozen screws holding those rods in place. I was awed by their courage. These girls were gutsy.

They were also patient. Today, these surgeries are equally long—surgeons can only move so fast. But the hospital recovery times are much shorter. The girls I cared for spent so much time in a post-op area two floors up that most came to us with their surgical dressings removed, and their sutures almost healed. They would spend a week or more with us, lying on their backs and doing little but wait for discharge. Today, post-op moves much faster. They're often standing on their second or third day and going home within a week.

As you might expect, caring for them meant embarrassment. By the time they came to us, these girls were off IVs and pain medications, so there was little to bring a nurse into their room. When I was first assigned to them on that fateful Monday morning, almost all their care fell on me. It resembled Christy or Min, but with four girls at once. Four, I felt on that first day, was at least three too many.

The summer heat made matters worse. Our climate control was far from perfect. My first winter on Hem-Onc, I added another item to my check list. The unit was exposed to winter on three sides, including the north, so rooms often dropped into the low sixties at night. When I entered a room, I'd grasp a little hand. If it felt cold, I'd make sure that boy or girl was better covered.

During that summer, Teens faced the opposite problem. Its rooms could get uncomfortably hot. For most patients that mattered little. Our halls weren't as hot as the rooms. When their rooms got miserable, they could walk about. But not everyone was that fortunate. Those who'd had serious surgery were confined to their beds. The boys, obsessed with privacy, endured that heat covered up. I felt sorry for them, but there was nothing I could do. I wasn't their problem. For the girls, as their primary caregiver I was their problem. Making matters even more complicated, their behavior could not have been more different from the boys. I saw that the first Monday morning I was assigned to their room on B cluster.

No top sheet was the first complication. Their room was on a corner that faced south and west. By late morning, with sunlight pouring in the windows, it was like an oven. Unable to get up, they kicked their top sheet down to the foot of the bed. That made sense. A sheet would have been almost unendurable.

The second complication lay in what they wore. Being girls, their dress was casual, thanks to our nearly all-female staff. Almost without exception, they didn't have any clothing under their gowns. That made sense. The time they had spent flat on their backs in post-op had taught them a lesson. Nature isn't fair. For girls, panties make bedpans a hassle. Leaving them off was also much cooler.

The third complication was the clincher. These girls were under orders to remain flat on their backs, occasionally turning on their sides to allow the skin on their backs to dry off. They could not sit up to cool off. Still worse, they dare not roll away from room's door, which often had teen boys walking by. That door had to stay open to permit air to circulate.

Do you get the picture? These four girls have nothing that would bring a nurse to their room. I'm expected to provide all their needs. If that wasn't enough, there was that terrible heat. They don't want a sheet. They don't want panties. Unable to sit up, they want to turn on their side to cool off. When they do that, the backs of their gowns flop open from top to bottom, usually toward where I was working with another girl. That was world in which they and I must live for several hours each day. Complicated, most complicated.

I saw what they were going through recently when I was hospitalized for the first time. My visit was also in the summer. In the daytime when my door was open, the room was cool. At night, with the door closed, the room became unbearably hot. My first night, I made a depressing discovery. Hospital beds aren't like ordinary beds. They're designed to be proof against body fluids. They don't breathe, so lying on one is like lying on plastic. I found myself doing what those girls did—rolling on my side when my back got hot and sweaty. I was as miserable as they and as desperate for relief.

That first morning with those girls, wild thoughts passed through my mind. Perhaps I could institute a rule that they must wear underpants when I was around. After all, I told myself, in a hospital underclothes are just clothes. There's nothing embarrassing about them. Then I realized that wouldn't work. The nurses would laugh and say that what these girls wore in their room was their business.

I also considered looking down at my shoes. That eliminated one problem, but would create another. I'd bump into things. Then those girls would laugh. They were the ones choosing to be so underdressed. Not wanting to look like a clown, I did neither.

To their credit, these girls were kind enough to give me a chance. They didn't act like our boys. None pulled up her sheets. None called for underclothes. None tucked in her gown. With the exception of one we'll call Miss Modesty, they even continued to roll on their sides. Why not? The alternative was far worse.

I was fortunate. Throughout my time at the hospital one aspect of my personality helped immensely. No matter how much stress I was under, I not only remained calm and thought clearly, I looked calm and in control. On Hem-Onc, my young patients and their parents sensed that and relaxed. These girls did the same. They probably thought I'd handled skimpily clad patients for years. While they relaxed, I scrabbled to figure out what to do.

Fortunately, the right ideas came quickly. First, as I had done with frightened little kids, I adopted the proper attitude and let that shape my behavior. This room was theirs, I reminded myself. I needed to enter like a guest and behave accordingly. With the kids on Hem-Onc, I reduced their pain as much as possible. With these girls, I would do all I could to reduce their embarrassment. It wouldn't be perfect, but it might be enough.

That led to my first guideline. I would come only when needed, typically when a girl pressed her call button. I would leave immediately afterward. No lingering. No lurking. I'd be like a pizza delivery boy at a slumber party. "Here's your pizza, now goodbye."

Unfortunately, by itself that meant little. As needy as these girls were, I still spent hours each day in their room. My second guideline made a real difference. Their room had one bed in each corner. As much as possible, I resolved that, when I was working with one girl, I'd face away from all the others. In one stroke, I'd reduced my presence in their room by 75 percent, giving each girl the equivalent of a private room. That eased their minds. Even when I was in their room, they were free to roll on their side.

Only one problem remained. I still had to come and go, and when I did there'd usually be at least one girl lying on her side. My third guideline dealt with that. It was impossible not to see the back of her gown flopped open, but it was possible to glance away quickly.

That mattered because these girls were watching me closely. My visits were almost the only entertainment they had. Years before, the hospital had raised enough money to put a small television next to every bed. But most were now broken and there wasn't enough money to replace them, in part because we provided free care to many kids. Watching me, each girl could see that I was glancing away from the others, but she couldn't see how I treated her. She had to take it on trust that I would do the same for her. That, I realized, was a key difference between teen boys and girls. The boys weren't willing to trust female staff and refused to yield even an inch of their privacy. These girls were willing to show flexibility, making my work easier.

Notice what those three guidelines taken together accomplished. On a typical day, I might spend over four hours with them. Without those guidelines, for all that time each girl would face a choice between misery and minutes-long exposure. With them, their exposure shrunk to a mere split-second. That left them free to cool off, and meant I didn't feel like a Peeping Tom.

Would those girls accept that for more than a day? I lived close to the hospital, so the next morning as I walked to work, I wondered if they would take my unspoken offer. They did, bless their wonderful girlish hearts. That is, all except Miss Modesty, who remained resolutely on her back, at least when I was in the room. That was fine. I could only give these girls better choices not perfect ones. Whatever they chose was fine. I constantly reminded myself that they had a right to their privacy, and that their cooperation was a courtesy for which I should be grateful.

They and I coped with that for seven long, hot days. Yes, my first assignment to these post-op girls had hit my long shift. To give nursing staff every other weekend off, our work schedule alternated seven days on with two off followed by three on with two off. Take my word for it, seven days of keeping those guidelines was exhausting. I felt like a stage actor in a difficult role who longed to see the curtain drop for the last time.

Near the end of those seven days, I received a surprise. I was helping a girl at the far end of the room and facing away as usual. Her bed happened to be next to Miss Modesty's. As I turned to leave, there was Miss Modesty on her side with her gown flopped open. I looked elsewhere, but as I walked away I wondered why she'd done that. She could not have missed me just three feet away. She must have decided to trust me—that and the heat. Yes, that heat was really bad. I can understand why they would do almost anything to cope with it.

I also took note of her change of mind, much like I took note of everything that mattered. It meant that a girl who'd been cautious could become more casual. Since the opposite was also likely to be true, I shouldn't presume too much on how a girl had acted in the past. Like the kids on Hem-Onc, I constantly collected observations and adjusted what I did. I fit care to the patient.

The result was an odd measure of success. Giving good care didn't hinge on eliminating all embarrassment. That was impossible. It hinged on how easily they and I could come up with a compromise that allowed them to relax. The existence of *some* embarrassing situations actually meant all was well. They and I were coping. Compared to the boys, where there was almost no embarrassment but much misery, the girls had it better.

With thought, you can find similar guidelines for your situation. Many hospitals avoid embarrassment issues altogether out of a fear that the resulting problems will be insoluble. The willingness of those girls to accept my patchwork guidelines suggests that patients will be flexible when given an opportunity. Most will meet staff half-way. So observe and discover what works. Clever tweaks help too. Later, I'll mention one based on the magical properties of an ordinary hospital towel—yes, a towel. And you thought it was just for bathing.

Would similar behavior by the female staff in the boys' room have improved matters? I'm not sure. Remember, I was fortunate. These girls were happy when I arrived and wanted to stay that way.

In that hot room, covering up meant misery. On the other hand, the boys were so unhappy even my male presence made little difference. They were resigned to their misery. Each multi-bed room had a culture that resisted change. When one girl checked out, the others modeled a relaxed attitude for the new one. In contrast, when one boy checked out, the remaining boys modeled staying well-covered, teaching the new guy to do the same. Both patterns were hard to break.

Would the boys' situation have improved if their nurses had created guidelines like mine? Maybe. Like reducing pain, lessening embarrassment typically does not interfere with good care. The specific guidelines might be different, but the core principle remains the same—do what you can and hope that's enough. Regard yourself as a guest in their space. Experiment and see what works.

Remember too, that the initiative to discover what worked for boys and men has to come from female staff. There was no way for me to discover guidelines for them, since they had no reason to mind my presence. With girls I would try something and note its impact. If it worked, I adopted it. If not, I tried something else. In return, they were marvelous, giving me the freedom to experiment and not appearing to mind my blunders, as long as I was trying. Unfortunately, with the boys nothing I did made any difference, so there was no way for me to learn. All I could do was observe. That said, I will offer one suggestion here. Elsewhere, I will explain the motivations that shape a teen boy's behavior. That may help.

Our teen boys were unhappy with having urine catheters placed by female nurses. Did that have to be nurse-only task, given how few men are nurses at some hospitals? Catheters aren't heart surgery. Male staff who aren't nurses could be trained to handle them. I won't pretend I'd enjoy that. But I'd be willing to learn for the sake of my patients. Remember, our teen girls could almost always have nursing procedures done by women. Expanding the pool of men who could do them would give our teen boys a similar freedom.

The idea might be extended to girls too. Pelvic exams done by male physicians are another troublesome area. The actual exam might still need to be done by a physician, male or female, but there's no reason why a female nurse couldn't handle the setup. Remember, patients like having their feelings considered. Easing their embarrassment a little may eliminate it altogether.

Seeing how quickly those three guidelines made a difference relieved me of my greatest worry. Based on past experiences, I'd been afraid that I would need to read each girl's mind and tailor my care specifically for her. That was difficult enough with one girl at a time. It would have been impossible with four at once. Therein lay madness. Fortunately, I found that the answer lay creating a overall climate in which these girls could feel safe. Helping them feel comfortable led to cooperation.

In a sense, this was repeating what I had learned on Hem-Onc. Working nights, I dealt with worried parents and frightened children. Once I showed them that I cared, that I was capable, and that I would be vigilant through those long nights, all went well. Parents slept, knowing I was watching over their child. The child would smile when I came in. I wasn't a monster. I was their friend, keeping the scary monsters away.

These teen girls were in a similar situation. I only needed to convince them that I wasn't a different sort of monster—a pervert on the prowl or a Peeping Tom lurking in the shadows. To do that, I showed I liked them. I also reduced their embarrassment to a minimum and gave them as many choices as possible.

I was amazed at how well that worked and later I'll explain why. In that first group, three girls traded a split-second of exposure for minutes of cool comfort. The other, Miss Modesty, was taken care of too. She only needed to stay on her back when I was around. Doing my best and giving as much choice as possible solved a problem that at first struck me as impossible. In fact, I came to enjoy working in that four-bed room. I found that I could handle four girls as easily as one—maybe even more easily, since each could learn from the others. Often that meant the shyer girls learned from the bolder.

Next, we'll examine another major embarrassment issue that I faced, one that would not go away—at least in my mind—quite as easily as those flopping gowns.

12. DRATTED BEDPANS

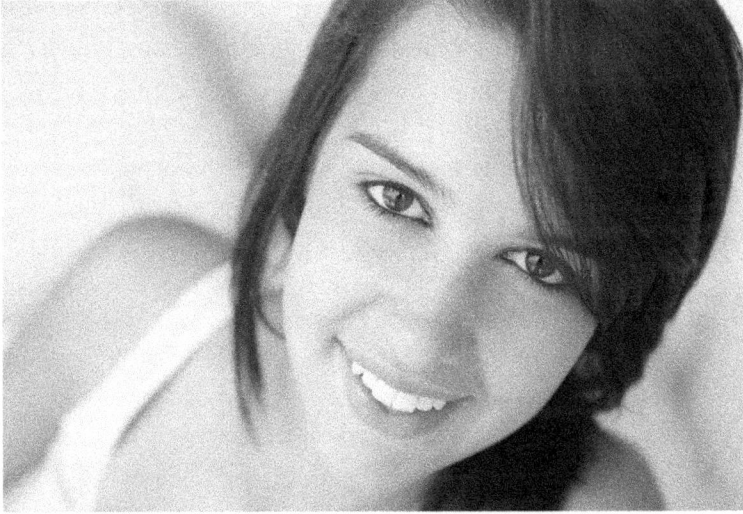

At first, I didn't understand why the nurse I was working with that day wanted my assistance. The patient was in his late teens and had been a paraplegic for years. He wasn't a frightened little child facing a procedure for the first time. There would be no need for me to hold him while she placed a urine catheter.

I went along anyway and, as I thought, merely stood there while she placed the catheter. It was then that I understood why I was there. She was uncomfortable about what she had to do and wanted me along for moral support.

A similar situation lay at the root of my second embarrassment crisis that summer. Unfortunately, I couldn't call on my nurse for support. That would have taken far too much of her time. I'd have to work this one out for myself.

Some say no good deed goes unpunished. That was certainly true in my case. Despite being new to caring for girls recovering from major surgeries, my quick response to their flopping gowns made me seem a seasoned professional. As a result, most trusted me with their bedpans. That's where events took a frustrating twist.

I liked my solution to the heat problem. It was elegant and sensible. My patients liked it too, since it reduced their embarrassment to almost nothing and solved a mutual problem. I hated bedpans though. I thought what we were doing was neither elegant nor sensible, so much so that I rebelled. I did nothing to encourage them to ask for a bedpan. I came and I went. I never asked, "Is there anything else you need?" If a girl wanted a bedpan, she'd have to speak up quickly. If she hesitated, I was gone. Yeah, tough. But like I said, I hated how we did bedpans. It was awful.

And no, it wasn't helping these girls that bothered me. I liked them and wanted them comfortable. I knew a full bladder was a misery and how rarely their nurse came around. For much of the day, I was their only hope for relief. When they asked, I quickly helped and didn't scowl. I didn't blame them for my unhappiness. But I still hated what I was expected to do. My sixteen months on Hem-Onc—where a single mistake might mean a child died—had made me a perfectionist. I could not tolerate anything less.

The problem arose because the first wave of post-op girls were experienced patients—perhaps too experienced. After a week or more in post-op, they knew the proper procedure for bedpans, having been taught by nurses in surgery two floors up. I knew it too. I'd placed untold bedpans under little kids and was extremely good at that. I could not have placed one more quickly or accurately. I took only a split second and never missed. Alas, that skill and quickness only meant more calls for bedpans. They knew that, as quick as I was, I couldn't be up to any mischief.

Much like that unfortunate nurse with her catheter, what didn't bother them did bother me, particularly how we were handling those bedpans. It struck me as all wrong. The standard bedpan procedure was designed by time-motion experts with hearts of stone. These girls would raise their knees and spread their legs wide. I'd look under their gown and place the bedpan in just the right place. While some bedpans don't require precise placement, ours—many so old the chrome-plating was wearing off—did. Get the placement a mere two inches off, and their sheets would need changing.

Nor am I the only one to feel this way. I've already mentioned how that nurse felt about a catheter. Read about the conflicting emotions that male medical students and residents go through when they learn delivering babies or pelvic exams and you'll sense my frustration. In my case, the situation was even worse. I wasn't dealing with a middle-aged mother of four or a street-savvy client at an STD clinic. No, these bedpan calls came multiple times a day and involved pretty girls in their mid- to late-teens. To get my reader's attention in *Hospital Gowns*, I was blunt. I call this posture "deliver my baby." It's the same that a woman in labor assumes. I hit them hard to make them think: "Do you really want to do this?" To drive my point home, I left out a critical detail.

From my perspective, what I was doing was no different from taking a temperature. Strange as it sounds, I saw nothing when I placed that bedpan—nothing at all. In fact, the same was true on the fewer occasions when I did the procedure for boys. Given my long practice, I unerringly hit the right spot without consciously seeing anything. Even more mysteriously, a moment later I knew whether a particular patient had undies or not. If she did, I'd need to pull them down before she could use the bedpan.

That placing without seeing was most mysterious, and no one was more surprised than me. What was going on? How had I acquired this strange power? Eventually, I concluded that knack was born while working nights with children. After Maria, I adapted how I treated boys and girls older than about six to take into account their budding modesty. Apparently, my subconscious decided to offer this assistance without bothering to inform me. Recently, I've read about why our subconscious does that. By blocking out sounds and sights that don't matter and emphasizing those that do, our minds help us cope with a world that would otherwise overwhelm us.

One illustration came from a soldier fighting in Europe during World War II, who described a battle he'd been in. Surrounded by loud explosions and rapidly firing machine guns, he heard none of that. Yet his attention was immediately riveted by the soft crunch of boots in the snow behind him. He turned just in time to shoot a German soldier sneaking up on him. His unconscious mind was filtering what he consciously heard. It knew that the usual sounds of fighting didn't matter and blocked them. It knew that soft crunch did matter and directed his attention to it.

That's what was happening with those bedpans. It explains why that unique knack existed from the start on Teens. It was already a well-honed skill. It explains why it worked equally well with boys and girls. It explains why it didn't filter out other embarrassing views. My subconscious hadn't made those a priority. It even explains why I didn't notice what was happening with those children at night. In darkened rooms, I was seeing so little, that I didn't notice I was seeing nothing. In brightly lit rooms on Teens, I couldn't miss what was happening.

Since these feelings are likely to apply to caregivers in other situations who may or may not have that mental block, I need to explain my frustration. I've already explained that, since I was seeing nothing, I had no objective reason to feel guilty. I had another reason I should have felt innocent—the girls themselves.

They weren't being forced into something they hated. I was as gentle as possible. Some girls never asked, waiting instead for the nurse or even asking me to get a nurse without explaining why. Since those vague requests almost always meant a bedpan, I could have lectured them on how busy the nurse was and how they should depend on me. I didn't. Later, I'll explain how that attitude put me on a collision course with the nursing administration.

As with flopping gowns, most girls did ask for my assistance, and that left me confused. None showed the slightest indication she minded the situation—not one. I know because I always watched for what upset these girls and shaped my behavior accordingly. That surprised me. Didn't they know their own anatomy?

Yes, I did realize that for many of these girls turning to me solved a pressing problem. I know how they felt. I experienced it myself not long ago when I was hospitalized with a greatly inflated bladder and two shut-down kidneys, the result of a swollen prostate. The instant I heard that diagnosis, I knew I wanted a catheter as soon as possible. I was rushed to a hospital room, where a male physician assistant assigned by a urologist saw my situation as the perfect occasion to teach three young, female nurses the procedure for a specialized catheter. Did I care? Not in the slightest. My bladder was about to explode, and my tummy was as hard as concrete. I wanted that misery gone. Nothing else mattered.

On smaller scale, these post-op girls felt much like I did. Comfort trumped modesty. But that only explains got-to-go-now situations where I was their only hope for relief. In *Hospital Gowns* I offered similarly placed girls a useful idea. Don't wait until your bladder is full, and you're forced to turn to male staff. Whenever a female staff enters your room, ask yourself if this would be a good time to ask for a bedpan. That's so obvious, it should have come to most of the girls I was caring for. Yet most turned to me even when they had alternatives. Embarrassment was not the only factor in their decision-making. These girls had other issues. One incident illustrates that.

I forget what sixteen-year-old Vivian's surgery had been, but with her right leg in traction, it wasn't a spinal fusion. The parents of post-op girls rarely visited, no doubt because these girls insisted, "I can handle this myself." Teens, both boys and girls, value their independence. But Vivian's parents had not only on visited her, they stayed long on one miserably hot afternoon. I could sense Vivian wanted them to leave, but I was on her parent's side. From how they were dressed, I doubt they had much money. This surgery cost them far more than they could afford. For all her independent spirit, they dearly loved their daughter.

When time came for them to leave, Vivian only waited a few seconds before calling on me to bring her a bedpan. "Me," I thought, "I'm a guy and that traction will make placing her bedpan slow and fussy. Why doesn't she ask her mother, who has changed her diaper times beyond counting?" Ah, but that was the exact point this girl wanted to make *to her mother.* She had not even waited for her mother to get out of earshot before calling on me—a guy. She wanted to stress just how independent she'd become. But her effort was badly mistimed. Since her mother was still within hearing, I called her back and let her handle the deed.

Are you sensing my frustration? Most of these girls had no problem with my handling their bedpans even when there were alternatives. Yes, I was amazingly quick, never missed, and always placed the bedpan before slipping down their undies, if any. All that reduced the potential for embarrassment somewhat. But when they asked, they didn't know I'd do all that. Yet they still asked.

Now is perhaps as good a place as any to bring up the "Dr. Mike syndrome." It refers to how these girls—bless their hearts—often regarded me. At the time, that left me both flattered and frustrated. Only recently have I began to understand what was happening. Elevating me far above my actual rank in the hospital's pecking order helped them cope with two issues that mattered to them.

For the first issue, put yourself into their heads. They've just experienced perhaps the most overwhelming event of their young lives. For some, it was a major surgery. For others, it may have been the diagnosis of a serious illness. They long for someone they respect, someone calm and mature, to assure them all will work out well. Yet what did the hospital offer? Our specialists were rarely around. The demand for their skills was too great. What those girls saw instead were typically overworked residents with dreadful social skills.

Then there was me, almost a decade older than those residents. I knew where I came up short. I had studied engineering not medicine. On Hem-Onc, I'd put an extraordinary effort into making myself skilled at one thing—spotting when a child with leukemia was in trouble. At that I was quite good. But that did me little good on Teens, where my patients had dozens of different illnesses. Often, I knew so little about a girl's illness, I had to look it up when she was admitted. My lowly status should have also been obvious. I was a drudge, taking care of bedpans, urinals, vomit and the like.

To my amazement, those girls did not see that. At times, they seemed to show me so much respect, I felt like saying, "Hey, I'm not your doctor. I'm just an assistant. Look at what I do—messy, yucky stuff."

Why did they give me such a boost? Because they saw in me what they wanted in their doctor, someone who had time for them and who was relaxed and confident that all would turn out well. Knowledge isn't everything. Strength also counts. Hem-Onc with had made me strong. I could pass that strength along to them.

Later, I'd realized I should have done more to repay their kindness. Many were told little and that's frustrating. I didn't have the expertise to know when a girl might go home, but I could read her medical chart and hint when she might do so. She'd be happy to hear from the news from her Dr. Mike. And if my prediction proved wrong? Well, don't forget that I wasn't a real doctor. I wasn't even pretending to be one.

The second issue contributing to my Dr. Mike status was the unusual relationship we had. As their sole male caregiver, these girls could not be neutral about me. They *needed* to trust me due to the potentially embarrassing assistance I gave. Watching me, they even *believed* I was worthy of their trust. But one question remained. What role was I playing in their care?

Yes, they knew I was nursing staff, but that didn't satisfy many. As a man, I didn't fit into their nurse box. That's not surprising. Almost all the hospital's nurses were women. As a result, many girls unconsciously placed me in their doctor box. "This is OK," they thought, thinking of something embarrassing. "He's like a doctor."

Yes, I was flattered, immensely so. But I was also frustrated because I felt they were trusting me more than I'd earned. They were giving me an A grade when I felt I did not deserve better than a C. With flopping gowns, I'd come up with the right guidelines to make their situation better, and I was proud of that. But with these dratted bedpans, the opposite was true. The procedure was dreadful, and I didn't know how to make it better. I felt like a failure.

Yes, I was fast with bedpans, but that counted for little. I'd learned that on nights, so children could get back to sleep quickly. That habit was so ingrained, I'm not even sure I could do a bed-pan placement slowly. Seeing nothing didn't ease my feelings either. My subconscious had done that rather than me. Besides, these girls didn't know about that. Unable to make sense of their trust, I felt insecure. If a girl had asked, "Why should I trust you, a guy, with my bedpan?" I wouldn't have had an answer. That bothered me.

I knew my feelings were out of kilter, so I tried to fix them. If my patients were comfortable, I told myself, why was I bothered? I knew the answer. I was bothered because I feared that they and I were living in a bubble that would later pop. Perhaps I was overcautious, but remember I not only liked these girls, I liked them all the more for trusting me so generously. Anyone who's worked in a hospital knows how wonderful trusting, cooperative patients are. Trust is the supreme compliment.

Remember too that I could walk in a few seconds from a room where the boys were cowering beneath their sheets—apparently lest a female nurse see their underwear—to a room were the girls could hardly be more relaxed and casual. It was natural for me to see one or the other as unusual. I had reason to worry that these girls might suddenly begin behaving like the boys, making me feel rotten.

Now imagine one of those girls, home a month and thinking back on those hot, boring days on the teen unit. Then a memory flashes into her mind. "Oh my gosh," she thinks, "what was I thinking when I called for that bedpan. What he must have seen... and not just once. This is so embarrassing."

Who would she blame? Would it be the nurses who taught her that procedure or me for cooperating? Most likely she'd blame herself for being so foolish. That's what I disliked. Time after time, my work meant placing these girls in embarrassing situations. I hated that some might later regret what they'd once accepted. Being hospitalized can distort our perspectives in ways that disappear when we return home. That bothered me.

It's not quite the same, but there's a situation close enough to illustrate that. While researching this book, I found an account on the website for the Scoliosis Research Society. Angelia, now a nurse working with scoliosis patients, was sixteen when she had a spinal fusion. Here's how she described what happened.

> I arrived at the hospital around 5 p.m. on the day before surgery. After blood tests and an explanation of the pre-operative process were completed, as a surprise my parents brought pizza and milkshakes for me and several of my closest friends. Later that evening, my doctor stopped by and said that he needed to take pictures of my back. He explained that he would use the photos to compare my back before and after surgery. The photos were taken in my underwear. One of the nurses stood with me as tears streamed down my face. To this day, it is one of the most humiliating moments of my life.

Angelia illustrates why I worried for these girls. I liked them. Willing and cooperative as they were, I didn't want to become a part of what might later become "one of the most humiliating moments" in their lives.

Fortunately, a answer would come, although not as soon as I would have liked. That's the next chapter.

13. Better Bedpans

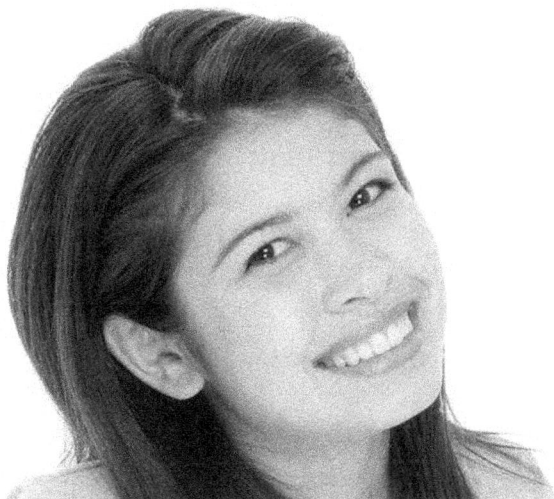

When I told a friend of mine, the mother of three charming preschool daughters, about my then-new book, *Hospital Gowns*, she understood what I meant. "After my third child was born in a hospital," she told me, "I gave up on feminine modesty." Circumstances, she was saying, can alter our perspective.

The early waves of post-op girls, with their numerous clinic visits over the years, followed by many days lying helplessly on their backs, resemble what she'd become as a mother of three. By the time that first wave came under my care, most gave every appearance of having given up on "feminine modesty." Faced with a choice between discomfort and exposure, almost all opted for comfort.

That made sense. In its advanced stages, scoliosis can move so rapidly, a patient's spinal curvature can change in mere weeks. For some, their surgeries came just in time. A short time later and they might have faced a lifetime of disability. These girls had good reason to be grateful, and some of their gratefulness was directed at me.

But their cooperation had a downside. It meant that I—and I alone—had to come up with ways to handle those embarrassing situations. That's why I scrambled to come up with those guidelines. On that first day they gave every indication of putting up with my presence even without them, but I wanted more. I wanted our situation handled with finesse. I wished these first girls had been motivated to be a bit more creative. Being trusted felt good, but having to do all the embarrassment management myself was exhausting.

Over the summer, I noticed a shift. As the surgeries became less serious, attitudes changed. For these later girls, their scoliosis wasn't yet in the danger zone. It merely couldn't wait until the next summer. Recall the contrast I drew between a desperate Tina, who felt she had to please our staff at any cost, and a grumpy Barb, who could care less whether I liked her. Of course, those girls remained friendly and cooperative despite their long, boring stay. But as the summer progressed, they displayed more initiative. That's why in *Hospital Gowns* I call them the "sensible girls." Sensible as in planning ahead and finding ways to lessen their exposure. Some wore undies, which made matters less complicated. Facilities must have done something about the air conditioning too, because the rooms became less sweltering.

Initially, the shift troubled me. The first girls were so casual, little embarrassed them. With these new girls, I wondered if they'd grow critical of my imperfect efforts. I imagined entering their room for the first time and seeing them pull up their sheets and squirm as they tucked their gowns underneath. Remember, that was how the boys handled their female caregivers. It could happen to me.

It never did. No doubt these girls wondered when I first took on their care. That was natural. But all were kind enough to give me a chance, and all went well. What they were doing before I arrived—which was being a bit more careful than the first wave of girls—they continued to do. None felt they needed to change because of me. That felt good. Though more cautious, they still trusted me.

I felt even better when I discovered that these new girls had what I sorely lacked—time to think. Long nights on Hem-Onc had given me time to work on problems. The hectic pace on Teens gave little time for thought. One demand quickly followed another. When I got home, I was too exhausted to think. That summer rush was particularly bad, since we were given no additional staff. Looking back, I remember incidents from then, but I have trouble recalling individual patients. Only later, as our workload eased, do I remember individuals. What I could not find time to do, these sensible girls did, coming up with practical solutions. I'll mention one in this chapter and another in the next.

I said I never consciously saw my bedpan placements. That's not strictly true. There was one occasion where my unconscious not only didn't block my vision, it actually called my attention to it, saying "You need to look at this." Think of that WWII soldier suddenly having his attention turned to that crunch in the snow behind him. This was like that.

What I saw were the girl's legs, but that wasn't what prompted my subconscious monitor. With only the her left hip visible, there was nothing in that replayed mental picture that was revealing. I realized why. To her credit, this savvy patient hadn't followed the procedure she'd been taught. With proper femininity, she'd kept her knees together and low, much like she was wearing a short skirt. Without realizing it, I'd followed her lead and placed her bedpan from the side, where the view was far more innocent.

In a instant, she solved my bedpan woes. No longer was I captive to those stony-hearted instructors. Her technique became the one I describe in *Hospital Gowns*. From that point on, my frustration with bedpans faded. Within a few weeks it was gone altogether. A procedure I hated became elegant and simple. Bedpans became mere drudgery, like most of my work.

Of course, learning that left me even more ticked off at the hospital. Being taught a bad technique, I realized, had kept me from seeing a better one. Bad techniques aren't just bad in themselves. They prevent us from seeing better approaches. That's particularly true in nursing, where a high priority is given to obeying orders. That's why hospitals must get what they teach right. In particular, they need to take into account opposite-sex issues and train staff to handle them. Everything done in a hospital doesn't need to be blindly unisex or designed for sheer speed. Two or three different techniques to achieve the same result are fine. Taking five seconds to do something rather than three will not bring an end to medicine. Staff are clever enough to learn several ways. Hospitals should be clever enough to teach them.

Hospitals should also ask for embarrassment feedback from patients. Indeed, I suspect that if they don't, patients will get fed up and force change. For small matters, they'll grade the hospital down in some other area, which may reduce third-party payments. That's because most patients are too embarrassed to mention embarrassment. For really bad incidents of the sort I discuss later, they'll file lawsuits, perhaps armed with secretly made smartphone recordings as evidence. With proper planning, those troubles can be avoided. Creative solutions should be encouraged, discussed, and rewarded.

The solutions those sensible girls taught me reaped benefits years later. Thanks to them, *Hospital Gowns* was born. What those girls taught, I decided to teach. Hospitals bureaucracies move slowly, so my first move was to write a book appealing directly to the girls. "By changing patients," I told myself, "I can change hospitals."

That seems to be happening. On one hospital's web page for girls getting scoliosis surgery, incoming patients were asking if it was acceptable to wear athletic shorts after their surgery. That gave me a warm glow, because that's what I'd recommended. Wear them, I told readers, and you can forget those revealing gown slits. You can even—if by wild chance your surgeon says yes—do cartwheels down the hall. To my delight, the hospital said athletic shorts were fine. We need a greater variety of hospital wear to ease the frustrations of those dreadfully revealing gowns.

Athletic shorts would also solve Min's problem. A large pair could have been slipped over her body cast, protecting her modesty and yet easily slipped down for toilet calls. Why didn't someone think of that? That has troubled me to this day. Sometimes we're blind to the obvious. Often it's a hospital system that, by not being creative itself, discourages creative thinking by others. But discouraging new ideas only leads to trouble, misery, and in Min's case to overwhelming fear. In contrast, encouraging one new idea leads to more in a virtuous circle.

In the next chapter we deal with another issue I faced that summer, one both I and my patients hated and for good reason.

14. Hated Linens

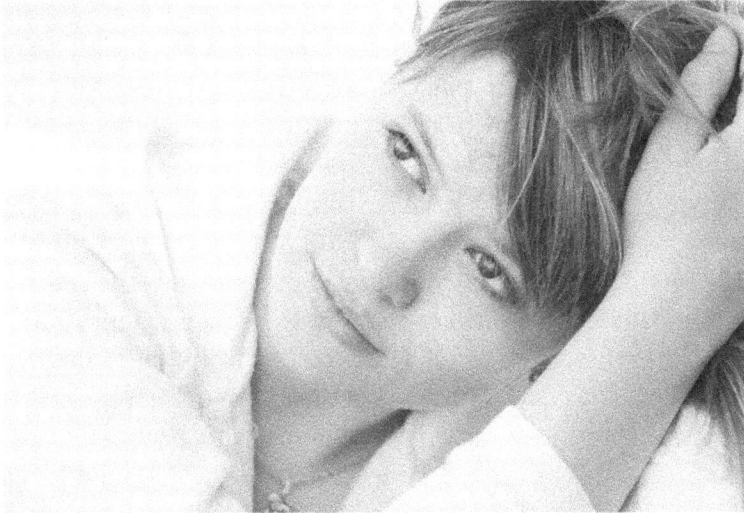

To my surprise those post-op girls were content with me as their caregiver. Flopping gowns were fine as long as I glanced away quickly. While I found bedpans frustrating, those who asked didn't mind, and those who did mind, didn't ask. That worked well enough. Once I found a better technique, my own anxiety faded.

But there was one situation that left these girls most unhappy. They hated it with passion and without exception. They'd clinch their teeth and stare ahead, as if I were a dentist about to drill. Distracting small talk did no good, and this one left them with no opt-out. I had to do it, and they had to endure it. It was really bad.

I'm talking about the linen changes that the hospital expected me, as the day-shift assistant, to do every three days come what may. They were as much a part of my job as bringing food trays. Since there's nothing inherent to linen changes that mandates doing them while a male staff is covering an all-female room (or vice-versa), it illustrates how rigid hospitals can be. Evening shift had women who had time for such work—more time than me in fact.

Let's look at where the trouble lay. With most patients, changing sheets was easy. I waited until they were up or asked them to get up for a few minutes. With those who'd had ordinary surgeries, it wasn't usually an issue. By the third day, they were up and often discharged. But linen changes were a serious matter for girls with spinal fusions. Their orders were inflexible. They must remain flat on their backs or briefly on their sides. My orders were equally firm, change those sheets while they lay there. In a seven-day stretch, I'd be expected to change twice. I couldn't deny their need for clean sheets either. Given the heat, by the third day those sheets really did need changing.

Ah, but when I did as ordered, the result was terrible. Removing the top sheet was easy—just pull it off. Often, they'd already kicked that down to the foot of their bed. But removing the sheet underneath meant trouble. I'd been taught to ask a patient to roll on her side away from me. I'd pull the old sheet from under the mattress, roll it into a long tube, and shove it next to her. Then I would tuck in a new sheet and place it, also rolled into a tube, next to her. Then she would roll over both sheets and lay on her other side. I'd go around, pull the old sheet off, and tuck in the new one.

That's efficient, but has a serious downside. Most of the time, a girl had nothing underneath. When she rolled onto her side, her gown would flop open toward an awkward-feeling me. These girls never tried to adjust their gown, although given how inadequate their gowns were, that wouldn't have done much good anyway. They just lay there feeling miserable. What they hated, I hated.

That confirmed what I'd suspected. Flopping gowns and placing bedpans hadn't provoked a reaction because a girl who found them embarrassing had options. I made sure of that. Those who went along wanted to do so. But linen changes didn't allow choice. Every third day, those sheets were to be changed. Even the most casual post-op girl hated it. Yet none objected. Hospital culture was so inflexible, I told myself, these girls cannot even say no to procedures they found painfully embarrassing.

Some might ask why these girls were so upset. After all, lying on their side to keep cool, which they did all the time, was little different from when they rolled on their side for a linen change. Why did they accept one situation in my presence but loathe the other? Ah, you've hit upon what I spent that first summer learning—how my patients *really* felt, rather than simply assuming what they *ought* to feel. Their feelings had a logic of its own, and I did my best to adapt, rather than dictate how they should feel.

I've already mentioned one reason why linen changes were so different. These girls had no choice. I began the summer doing my best to give them options. I concluded that for many being able to avoid a situation made them more willing to accept it. Choice creates trust and trust brings cooperation. That's the good cycle. Lack of choice creates discomfort and resistance. That's the bad cycle.

You see that in the dramatic difference between our girls and boys. Thanks to how Teens was staffed, our girls always had a choice about their bedpans. If calling on me was too much, there was a nurse who was always female. That helped them relax. Except for when I worked on their cluster, the boys didn't have that choice. Their nurse and assistant were women. That explains their sulking.

Let's be blunt. All the efforts those boys made—gowns tucked in and sheets pulled up despite the heat—were devoted to one purpose, keeping our female nurses and assistants from seeing the underwear that they, without fail, were wearing. They didn't want that exposure even for a split-second. Silly as it sounds, that was it. Remember too that the boys had it much easier. Urine voids weren't as complicated as for girls. For boys, all our female staff needed to do was hand them the urinal stored under their bed. Yet they balked at even that.

The girls illustrated the opposite. They cooperated even when they might have said no. Rather that sulk, they were doing their best to befriend me. But with those linen changes, they were clearly unhappy. It was too much. I'd have to be blind not to see that.

There's a boy-girl distinction that may help us understand this difference. When patients were first able to get up and move about in their gowns, an issue came up. The nurses I worked with were quite tolerant of patient undress in rooms, but they considered it "inappropriate" for patients to wander about our halls with the back of their gowns popping open. In practice that only had meaning for our girls. The nurse and I would often catch them about to leave their room with their gown back unpinned and insist on pinning it up. That happened so often, I carried safety pins in a pocket of my tunic just for them. But as best I recall, we never had to pin up a guy's gown. They always took care of that themselves, typically by never leaving their room clad only in a gown. When it came to modesty, the two sexes were different. Our boys were more modest.

What lies behind those differing attitudes might be called the "oops moment." When it comes to clothing, guys and girls grow up in different worlds. Men's clothing emphasizes size and strength—the padded shoulders of coats for instance or bulky, loose-fitting pants. Only rarely does it expose anything. In their everyday life, men don't need to worry about something—say their underwear—being exposed. Placed in a hospital where such exposure is common, they don't like it. It seems unnatural, so they rebel.

Not so with women. From their early teens on, women grow up in a more risqué world. Their fashion is driven by what part of a feminine body will be tantalizing almost exposed this year. Skirt hemlines move up. Blouse necklines move down. Even when women wear pants, they're often low-rise or extremely tight. If anything, teen girls, in their efforts to compete with other girls, push those 'almost exposed' limits further than their mothers, hence that perpetual mother-daughter conflict.

Here's an example. I live close to a state university and walk around its campus every weekend. On a recent walk I was surprised to see dozens of young women, all coming from the same direction and spreading out across campus. Asking one confirmed what I thought—it was sorority rush. I joked with another that their sheer number made me feel like I was visiting a woman's college.

Given that it was rush, I wasn't surprised that all wore colorful summer dresses. Later, I realized I'd seen confirmation of the point I'm making here. No guy wears clothing that is risqué on windy days. If it'd been gusty that day, more than a few of those girls would have found those light skirts blowing in their faces. Why accept that? Because those dresses make them look pretty—very pretty indeed. For that, they're willing to accept a little embarrassment. On Teens, girls even anticipated that by doing what no boy ever did, bringing their cutest undies from home. If their undies were seen, apparently these girls wanted them to be pretty. Avoiding embarrassment was but one motivation among many.

That's why, even before they came to us, these girls had faced far more "oops moments" than our boys. They'd learned to be phlegmatic about brief slips. A split-second of exposure was, for most, no exposure at all, or at least not one they worried about. That explains their attitude toward flopping gowns and bedpans. Those were oops moments. As long as they trusted me and the time was brief, all was well. Unfortunately, linen changes were not oops moments. That tolerable split-second of exposure became a painful minute or more. That was too much, hence their great discomfort—and mine.

I would have been delighted if they're responded to linen changes by saying "No," and perhaps even insisting, "I would rather the woman who works evenings did this." That would have given me an excuse to do nothing. Alas, not one did, probably out of kindness to me. They knew this was something I was supposed to do and didn't want to hurt my feelings. Instead, I had to be as kind to them as they were to me. Given the stern work ethic the hospital imposed, I wasn't supposed to evade linen changes. But since these girls weren't rebelling, I rebelled for them. I still did linen changes for other patients, meaning those who could get up. But I managed not to find time for these bed-bound girls. That wasn't hard. Remember, we were very busy that summer. I could fake being too busy for that.

There were occasions when the nurse I was working with noticed what I wasn't doing and persuaded a woman assistant from a different cluster to help me. My co-worker would take one side of the bed while I took the other. That halved a girl's exposure, but made no difference. Half of terrible was still terrible.

Although I didn't realize it at the time, I was fortunate. Our regular head nurse—more about her later—was away on leave. The nurse who was substituting was one of the sweetest in the hospital. She never raised a word of objection to my Great Linen Rebellion. I got away without a scratch.

Of course, from time to time my work load would slack off enough I'd find myself with nothing to do but change linens. That was particularly true near the end of the summer, when I might have only one or two bed-bound girls to care for. In such a situation, I couldn't stand around doing nothing.

Fortunately, that turned out OK, as one clever girl showed me a better way. Rather than roll on her side like she had been taught, she bounced on her bottom to the other side of the bed, taking care to hold down her gown. All the other gown changes had left me feeling awkward, standing there with no place to look. What she did was so cute, I enjoyed watching. Thanks to her, I now had a better way to handle bed linens. Alas, by then it was late summer and patients like her were rare.

Now is perhaps a good place to tell the real secret to doing linen changes. It's that magical towel I mentioned earlier. All I needed to do was bring a large towel with the other clean linen and place it across a girl's hips. Presto, when she rolled on her side, she was well-covered. It really is magical, making what ought to be hidden remain hidden. That would also teach these girls, so afraid of offending me, that it I wouldn't feel a bit bad if they covered up.

Towels would have also been handy in other situations. One particularly bothered me. With girls who'd had spinal fusions, I gave up checking the long incision that ran down almost their entire back. My excuse was that, since their dressings were removed before they came to us, a check wasn't necessary. I knew I was kidding myself. Lying with their backs continually damp and warm might trigger a belated skin infection. Yet every time I thought about doing such an inspection, I decided, "No, I'm not going to ask these girls to do that. That would be even worse than a linen change." A towel would have solved both problems.

Looking back, it's clear I wasn't thinking clearly. I was already using a towel with another procedure—a spinal tap. For it, patients had to lie on their sides, curled up and exposing the small of their backs. From their front, I pinned them down at their upper legs and waist. Then a resident working from behind inserted a needle into their lower spine. On my own, I decided to make that less unpleasant by using a towel as a surgical drape. That seemed to make them more comfortable. If you ask why I didn't extend that to linen changes, I don't know, other than that I was too tired to think well.

But enough of these negatives and workarounds. In the next chapter I'll describe a spectacular success, one that to this day still amazes me. It also offers a fascinating insight into the hearts of these marvelous patients. They never ceased to astonish me. That's why I loved caring for them.

15. Beautiful Smiles

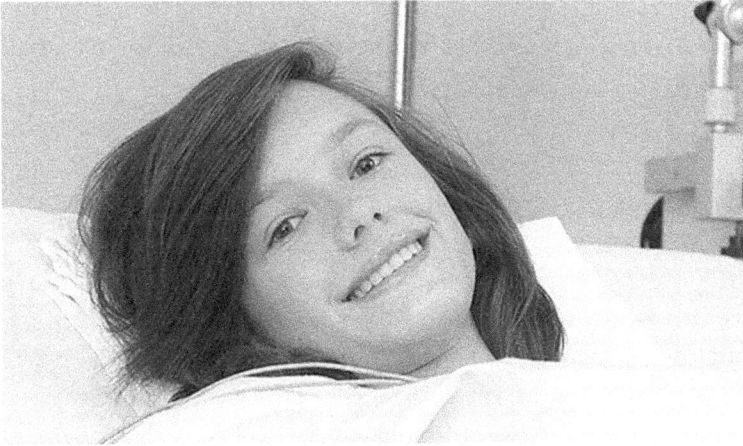

The gym at my high school was adapted from a large, World War II-era Quonset hut. The modifications to make it serve that purpose meant that not every part was used as originally intended. Showers, for instance, might have a row of clear windows in the pre-fab steel walls. That's not something you often see.

One day in the seventh grade, as I was waiting at the corner of the gym for the bell to ring, a girl in my class spoke to me from behind heavily painted-over windows. When I answered, I discovered she was showering after her PE class. I never understood what prompted her to start our conversation, but I did find it memorable. What healthy 13-year-old guy would forget talking to one of the prettiest girls in his class as she showered, covered with nothing but soap bubbles?

Caring for hospitalized teens had much the same flavor, with that painted-over window being replaced by those gowns. In both cases something risqué was going on, but the situations on the teen unit were far more complicated. My seventh-grade friend knew that there was no risk of being seen behind those painted windows. Not so our teen boys, in the case of female nursing staff, or teen girls, in my case. For both, embarrassment was a real possibility.

The result was dramatic. The boys, feeling that they'd lost control of something that mattered, turned to the flight side of fight or flight and withdrew. Put their deeds into words and they were saying, "Get lost. Leave me alone. I don't want you around because you embarrass me." That's why I've tried to go easy on the nurses I worked with. They had it much tougher than I.

The girls, seeing their circumstances more in terms of tend and befriend, turned to befriending, and I was obviously the one they should befriend. To my surprise, that, coupled with their trust of me, often put a spirit of girlish adventure into their hearts, much like my seventh-grade friend's decision to talk with me. Put their deeds into words and they were saying, "See, I'm being helpful and cooperative. Now will you please embarrass me as little as possible." That made my work easier, and for that I'm most appreciative.

Keep in mind a critical distinction that made my work with these girls easier. The boys wanted to feel in control of all that was happening, and there's nothing a hospital is less willing to relinquish than the ability to dictate what patients do and have done to them. That I could not change. Since I was never able break down their resistance, it's hardly surprising that our nurses, with the additional complications of embarrassment, could not.

On the other hand, our girls were much more cooperative. I imagine that for many their only real interest in controlling their care came when I showed up and embarrassment became an issue. Fortunately, since I was their sole problem, I could offer workable solutions. I could do my best to lessen their embarrassment and, when possible, leave them with the option of avoiding even that. That left them feeling safe.

You've heard of my first success with those flopping gowns, followed by what I saw as failures with those dratted bedpans and the universally hated linen changes. With that latter two, my hospital training was useless. Answers came from watching my patients. I'll finish out this description of that fateful summer with an over-the-top success. Be prepared to be astonished.

To the best of my memory, I don't recall a single case where a teen guy vomited onto his gown. They had it easy. Their summer surgeries typically involved legs or knees that'd been injured in sports or motorcycle accidents—the usual results of masculine risk-taking. Although stuck in bed, they could sit up and that put their mouth higher than their stomach where it belongs.

Unfortunately, that was not true for girls with back surgeries. Ordered to lie flat, eating was difficult. Even worse, with their mouths at the same level as their stomachs, they often spit up. Usually just after lunch, a call light would go on, and I would discover a girl whose gown was covered with vomit—sticky, smelly, and acidic. She was upset at what she'd done, and I'd assure her that it happened all the time. Now ponder the quandaries she and I were in.

First came the need to act quickly. The hospital believed in cleanliness almost to a fault. That icky gown had to be changed fast and doing so was my job. The nurse would be most unhappy if I called on her for that. Day-shift nurses were overworked and avoiding embarrassment wasn't a priority. Remember what I said about the 'staff are not male or female' dogma. Like it or not, I had to take their attitudes into account. Patients came and went, but nurses remained. I had to keep them happy.

Second came the potential for embarrassment on a grand scale. Remember what I said about many girls deciding panties were too much bother? That was even more true with bras. Except for sad little Tina, who'd just arrived, bras were never worn. And no, I didn't yank up their gowns to look. That was easy enough to see from the slit in the back of their gowns. To do my job, I needed to know just how much each girl had on. The less she wore, the more careful I needed to be.

In *Hospital Gowns* I suggested that, if it made them feel more comfortable, my readers should wear underpants or, even better, athletic shorts. That's a good idea. Despite what many nurses believe, slipping down undies beneath a gown to use a bedpan isn't that much trouble. Good male staff won't mind, and the feelings of the creeps doesn't matter—as I repeatedly reminded those girls. Do what makes you comfortable, I told them, and don't worry about staff. They'll adapt. In fact, wearing athletic shorts is an good way to signal to observant nurses that you're not that into embarrassment. They'll notice and adjust what they do.

But bras are different. In *Hospital Gowns* I didn't attempt to persuade readers to wear them because I knew they wouldn't listen. In a hospital, abandoning that pesky item makes sense. Bras are hot and uncomfortable, particularly when you're confined to bed. For all their flaws, gowns do protect feminine modesty there. Instead, I suggested that my readers keep a bra, a sports bra, or even a swimsuit top near their bed. If staff need to do a chest exam—not that common with teens—a well-prepared girl can ask for a moment alone to dress better.

Now back to that first unfortunate girl with her messy gown. With not a scrap of clothing underneath, what were she and I to do? I had drawn the curtain around her bed as soon as I saw the problem. But that would only shield her from the eyes of the other girls. I was the real issue. Fortunately, my training had *not included* this dilemma, and by now you know that was good. I had nothing to unlearn. Watching how these girls responded, I'd do my best and discover what worked.

I was fortunate in another way. Remember Christy, the gentle girl I cared for on Hem-Onc who died of a brain tumor on her fifteenth birthday? We're now at the point I said would be explained later. She was even more helpless than these girls and, for reasons I never understood, would occasionally vomit on her gown in the middle of the night.

The first time, I took a chance that depended on her trusting me. Knowing how little she could do, I placed a new gown alongside her messy one. Then I switched the two, taking care to look nowhere but in her eyes. She was delighted. Since the technique was simple, elegant, and utterly devoid of embarrassment, I liked it too.

So when that same situation first arose on Teens, I decided to take a chance, although with a little fear and trembling. Over those nights, Christy had ample time to learn to trust me. This post-op girl had less opportunity, so I would be asking a lot of her. Making matters still more complicated, Christy and I were in a dark room. This girl's room was brightly lit. Not knowing what else to do, I plunged ahead, taking care to look deeply into her eyes.

I was amazed. Not only did it work, after the gown exchange, an enormous smile broke out on her face. I could understand a mere grudging acceptance of the inevitable, but how could I explain that smile? Why did the most potentially embarrassing of all circumstances make this girl so happy?

Over that summer, I faced that situation over and over. Each time, I expected the girl to cross her arms, glare, and say, "Don't touch my gown, you pervert. I want a woman." That never happened. Instead, each time I saw a face lit by that astonishing smile.

At first, I was mystified. Eventually, I understood. When I arrived, they were carefully watching this bearded guy who'd blundered into their life, wondering if he could be trusted. I was, after all, the most important person in their lives that day. They needed me, but had reason to be suspicious. Hospitals are intrusive and guys more so. For all they knew, I might rush up and scatter what little clothing they had on for some nefarious purpose.

By early afternoon, each girl had been watching me for a few hours to several days. That proved enough. They had decided that maybe—just maybe—I could be trusted. That's when their befriending kicked in, and why they cooperated with what must have seemed a risky way to rid themselves of a messy gown. Their smile came when their trust proved justified. "My befriending has worked," they thought, overjoyed as only a helpless hospital patient can be. From their girlish perspective, that was a wonderful success. They had trusted and I hadn't peeked even for an instant. Call that "virtual privacy" if you want. What mattered to those girls wasn't what was exposed but what was seen.

Yes, I have trouble imagining one of our teen boys behaving like that. In a similar situation, a nurse could consider herself fortunate he didn't hit her. As always, the guys were different. With a guy, the best advice I can give is to draw the curtains, give them a clean gown, and let them change it themselves. They'll like that. Changing yourself is masculine. Being changed by others is for babies.

To make these girls' responses more intriguing, I didn't make their cooperation easy. I never explained in advance. I just plunged ahead, for some reason confident all would go well. Why didn't I tell them what I was going to do? I never asked myself why, but I can guess. Suppose I'd said, "Listen, I'm going to place a new gown alongside your messy one. Then I'm going to swap the two, but don't worry, for those few seconds, I'll be looking you into your lovely eyes. I won't see a thing." Would that have been better? Maybe. But there are reasons why a silent approach might be best.

First, explaining in advance would have taught these girls to trust what I said. I wanted them to trust me. By saying nothing, I encouraged them to assume that I'd always do my best for them. Given how long they and I would be together—often for a seven-day stretch—that mattered. If a more complicated situation arose, say a messy bout of diarrhea, they would still trust me.

Second, Christy taught me that, where there's trust, explaining isn't necessary. Actions are what matters. With these girls, when I did the right deeds, they relaxed and all went well. Remember, I never told the girls in that hot room about my three guidelines. I simply followed them, and they responded. They were excellent observers. The same was true with bedpans. Rather than offer explanations, I was quick and flawless. With linen changes, I simply quit doing them. Explaining something that stupid was pointless. Gown changes were another case where deeds were better than words.

Third, I knew words had not been needed on Hem-Onc. Most of my leukemia patients were so young, they understood little about what I did. Why did I put a little plastic stick in their armpit? Why did I place the cuff that squeezed around their arm? Why did I fiddle with that strange beeping box on a pole? All that was beyond their understanding. Instead, they simply believed I was looking after them through those long nights. That was what mattered. When I transferred to Teens, I did the same. I let my deeds speak for me. All in all, that worked quite well.

Besides, I liked their beautiful smiles.

16. Traveling Companions

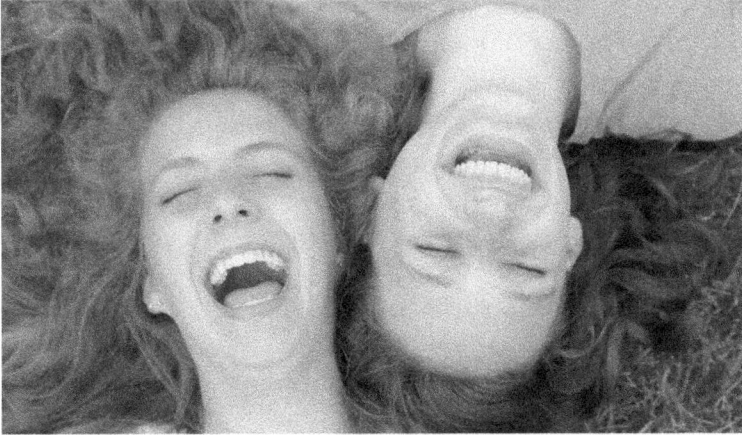

Earlier, when I described the unhappiness of our post-op boys, I suggested that their woes came from not being allowed to express their growing manhood, something they had good reason to be sensitive about. We expected them, in Shakespeare's words, to lie "a-bed" thinking themselves "accursed" and holding "their manhoods cheap," even as they battled an illness or recovered from a major surgery. We wanted passive, obedient patients—not a role easily assumed by teen boys, least of all those whose hospitalizations often came from adolescent risk-taking. Unable to do anything they regarded as manly, they withdrew into sullen silence. In literary terms, they were unhappy knights, leaving the dragon slaying and princess rescuing to others. We could have done better.

What about our post-op girls? Did they share similar feelings of unhappiness? After all, they were in almost identical situations. Not that I could see. They seemed unperturbed by their helpless state. Unlike our teen boys, most accepted at least some of the embarrassing situations that arose. Why were they so different?

Perhaps some experiences I had a few years before that can shed light on their attitude. They involve women, most just a few years older than these girls, who were facing sexual harassment when I met them while touring Europe.

I visited Berlin during a cold, damp November. When the time came to leave, I went to a station to take a train back to West Germany. This was during the coldest years of the Cold War. Although in West Berlin, the station was run by the East German government with the usual communist indifference to people. There was no heated waiting area and not even a place to sit in the lobby. Resigned to my misery, I sat on the floor to wait two hours for my train.

A few minutes later, a dark-haired girl of about twelve sat down next to me. With twenty feet of wall on either side of us, Miss Little obviously wanted to be with me, and I soon realized why. The station was in a rough part of the city. Some of those passing through made me, a grown guy, nervous. They must have been terrifying to her. I resolved to make sure no one hassled my little friend.

My attempts at conversation got nowhere. I knew almost no German, and Miss Little knew no English. She was content to sit next to me, watching me read. When the loudspeaker announced my train, I stood up to leave. In an instant, she flitted into the night like a frightened bird. "Her home life must be really bad," I thought, "to send her out on a night like this."

Notice what had happened. She and I had never met before and had no language in common, yet we understood one another perfectly. She was saying, "I need your help on this scary night," while I responded with protection. You don't need words to convey human motivations that basic.

As winter descended on Northern Europe, I moved further south, chasing after warmth. There I discovered to my delight that meeting American girls had become remarkably easy. In Northern Europe, as the guy I had to take the initiative. In Southern Europe, they'd hover nearby for a few minutes, then approach me. Shortly after that, a connection was made, and we'd travel together until our paths parted. The only exception came in Vienna, where my efforts to shepherd four girls came to an end when they deserted me for four boys. They were more than I could handle anyway.

Why was there this difference between Northern and Southern Europe? I can offer an illustration. Two American girls I met on a Spanish train had canes strapped to their packs. Since they had no problem walking, I wondered why until they explained. The canes were to shove away unwelcome advances by pesky Spanish males—I won't call them men. Those two girls would be the first in a series of traveling companions. By this point, I'd spent some three months living out of a backpack. I was tired of museums and eager for charming companionship. Every time I had feminine company, they would explain their hassles from the local males in this, the boorish part of Europe. People who stay in five-star hotels may claim all cultures are equal. Those who travel on tight budgets know better, particularly if they're young, pretty, and female.

Almost always, there was a short period during which I was auditioned. At Pompeii, a young woman quietly followed me from exhibit to exhibit until she decided I could be trusted and began a conversation. After that, we spent the afternoon roving Naples, using her Spanish as a substitute for Italian. Miss Naples taught me something. Judging by her conversation, she was quite experienced in a worldly sort of way. Yet she found the Italian males as irritating as the most sheltered of the other girls. A creep is a creep.

With my rail pass about to expire, I wrapped up my European travels by heading to Brindisi at the heel of the Italian boot, where I could catch a ferry to Greece. Eating lunch in a park, the familiar game played out. Two American girls on vacation from a German language school sat on a bench next to mine and, after a few minutes, struck up a conversation. I'd passed yet another audition.

The last night before the ferry left, those two girls and I were eating in a cafe when a woman joined us. Miss Athletic was an impressive six-foot-four tall with the broad shoulders of a football quarterback. She could take care of herself, which made the story she told hilarious. At about the same time those two girls were attaching themselves to me, an Italian guy she called "the little monkey man" forced his attentions on her. Claiming the hostel those girls and I stayed in our first night was closed, Monkey Man persuaded her to stay with him. We laughed. She had little to fear. If he'd misbehaved, she could have tossed him against a wall.

Unfortunately, most girls weren't like Miss Athletic. Creeps like Monkey Man were ruining their lives. Traveling meant an exhausting risk assessment made all the worse by the fact that they knew almost nothing about a country or its people. "Where will it be safe to stay tonight?," they had to ask. "Is this neighborhood OK to walk through? Is it too dark now or will it be too dark when I come back? Will this night train be safe?" The questions went on and on.

Ah, but these girls had an answer The solution to a bad guy, they realized, was a good one. Almost all creeps are cowards. That's why they target unaccompanied women. A male companion intimidates because they can't predict what he'll do. Yes, he might prove a coward like Mr. Chicken. But he might be skilled in martial arts or simply stand his ground bravely. Even the masculine bent to violence serves a good cause here. Given sufficient reason, some men can shift in a flash into a cold, calculating, pitiless use of force. "Mess with her," they decide, "and you'll end up so mangled, you'll spend a month in the hospital." Creeps know and tremble. That's why my presence sent them flying. I didn't have to do anything, because they didn't know what I might do. Deterrence works.

If psychologists take note of this phenomena, they might give it a dreadful name like "asymmetric male-female bonding." They need not do that. There's an well-established term for it—chivalry. Think brave knights, pretty princesses, sharp swords, fiery dragons, and the like. It may be politically incorrect to say so, but there's something in many women that makes them like being protected by a man they trust. That feels good. The masculine parallel is also true. There's something about the right men—meaning not creeps and predators—that likes the respect given to the chivalrous.

Ah, but there was one risk these girls could not avoid. That involved finding that good guy. Imagine a countryside where the predators are wolves, the chivalrous are sheep dogs, and sheep are the victims. The sheep are obviously better off with the sheep dogs, but how can they tell the difference? Both wolves and sheep dogs are members of the same species or, in this case, the same sex.

That explains our subtle dance. First, I had to wait for them to initiate contact. Creeps were invariably pushy, so I had to show I wasn't. By letting them make the first move, I demonstrated I'd let them break away. That reduced their risk. The second step happened about an hour or so later when their feelings shifted from wondering to trusting. When that happened, our separate travel plans became mutual. A girl would talk about what she'd like to do, but leave the details to me. Security became my department.

To give an illustration, at a hostel in Jerusalem's Old City a European girl mentioned she'd like to attend a concert by a Danish orchestra that evening. I offered to take her, and she accepted. I called ahead to arrange tickets and planned how to get there. That was no small task. Jerusalem is one of the world's most dangerous cities. City buses had a bad habit of exploding. I also took note of the time we took to get there. The hostel locked its door at 10 p.m., so we'd need to leave early to get back in time.

Notice the differing roles. By partnering with me, Miss Europe gained *more* freedom. Going to that concert by herself was risky. Paired with me, she could do more. What did I get? Certainly not more freedom. As a young guy with little money, I could roam at will. Pairing meant added responsibility. I had to look out for her as well as myself, scanning ahead for trouble as we walked. What I got in return was something I appreciated—her trust. Companionship, even if only for a single evening, made both our lives more enjoyable. It established one of the most deep-seated of all human relationships, a bond of trust between men and women.

Recall the two girls in Spain who'd been terrified by a night on a crowded train. They'd bought canes, but knew a guy like me was better. Traveling to Madrid, I was alone in a train compartment with my favorite of the two, the slender Miss Spain. Still sleepy from that terrible night, she curled up next to me and fell sound asleep. Those creeps had scared her. I made her feel safe. That's trust.

Miss Naples offers another example. As we saw the city, she told me about the rotten Italian males who would have been bumping up against her if I wasn't there. I could have said, "Yes, but sightseeing together we're bumping into one another all the time. What's the difference?" "You're different," she would have said. Notice this was from a woman who, when she wasn't talking about local creeps, told me about the men she'd slept with. I never figured out if she was trying to impress or seduce me. I was just glad I'd already told her I'd be leaving on an early evening train.

My time with the two girls in Brindisi was similar. The evening of the day we met, I found them a place to stay in a youth hostel, walking them there after dark. I was particularly concerned about one of them. Soft and gentle, Miss Delicate was so pretty she made my head spin. She'd grown up in an wealthy community with tree-shaded streets named after Ivy League universities. Sheltered all her life, her last few days of travel had plunged her into horrors that had made even the tough-talking Miss Naples furious. I did my best, and she responded with a trust so intensive it scared me. "Don't trust me so much," I felt like saying.

While working on Teens, I don't recall drawing analogies to my experiences traveling, but they must have shaped what I did. My first morning working with a new group of girls, there was an audition during the initial hour or so. That I understood.

What I didn't understand with those first post-op girls was the distinction they made between bad and good guys. I didn't realize that, if I made it into the latter category, all would go well. I thought that at best they would see me as harmless and thus neutral rather than good. To achieve that, I scrambled to reduce their exposure as much as possible. At least they will find me tolerable, I thought.

Only later did I realize what was happening. Those girls were thinking much like the napping Miss Spain, the sightseeing Miss Naples, and trusting Miss Delicate. By doing my best to keep their exposures brief and freely chosen, I was a good guy. Even those linen changes, as much as they hated them, were endured in silence. For them, trust was key. Trust made the difference between comfort and discomfort—much as it did with those girls traveling.

Did guys who were traveling share corresponding experiences? Yes and no. Yes, similar things did happen to us. But no, our responses were different. That's a key distinction to keep in mind.

One came while I was in the Scotland attending the Edinburgh Festival. Since I had a Britrail pass that covered all my rail travel, rather than pay for expensive housing in Edinburgh, I was staying at a youth hostel in Glasgow and making the forty-some mile trip back and forth each day.

One evening, as I was returning to the hostel, I saw six young women coming toward me on the sidewalk ahead. They'd obviously been drinking and were singing these lines from the popular musical, *My Fair Lady*:

Girls, come and kiss me;
Show how you'll miss me.
But get me to the church on time!

That first line proved a warning. When they reached me, I found myself surrounded and facing a demand that I kiss the bride-to-be. Telling myself, "When in Glasgow, do as the Glasgowians," I did.

I could take that easily, because I was a guy and felt in no danger, even out-numbered six-to-one on a darkening street in a city I knew little about. They were women. I was a man. Why worry? That's how we think as men—most of us anyway. We rarely regard women as physical threats.

Ah, but have six obviously drunk guys making similar demands of a lone young woman on a dark street in a city she doesn't know, and you'd have a different situation wouldn't you. It might be OK, but it might not. That difference makes a big difference.

Here's what that means. Not seeing any necessity, men don't develop the skill to cope with threats from women. Why should they? Physically, they can handle whatever comes. Whether a woman means them good or ill means little. They are still stronger.

Ah, but what happens when a major surgery leaves men poorly clothed and dependent on female nurses and assistants for their every need? Unable to think, "This is a good woman. I see she can be trusted. She won't harm me," they withdraw. They're facing a problem their life experiences have left them ill-equipped to handle. The result was disaster.

Compare that to women. From their early teens, they know men pose risks and learn, most of them, to observe and determine if a particular man is good or bad. Good men they trust. Bad men they don't. Unable to use physical strength, they rely on carefully honed feminine intuition to spot the differences between the two.

That's how those post-op girls dealt with issues that make kissing a stranger seem trivial. While our boys were sulking, those girls were watching me. It's also why I came to like caring for four at once. The more that happened, the more they could observe. It's also why I used curtains around their beds only when absolutely necessary. I *wanted* them to watch me work.

Bedpans didn't require a curtain, so when a bold girl became the first to ask for a bedpan, the others could see that went quickly and smoothly. That eased their minds. Drawn curtains would have dealt with flopping gowns, but only by adding to the stifling heat. Not using them meant they could see my efforts to create virtual privacy. Again, they saw and learned. Each girl, bless her heart, assumed that, if I looked quickly away for other girls lying on their sides, I'd do the same for her. Our girls learned to trust by watching. Our boys did not do that. They valued power and control.

Drawn curtains made linen changes worse. No girl could see and draw assurance from how I handled the others. Facing away, no girl could see how I was handling her either. Indeed the whole procedure was so stupid, not seeing was impossible. That's where a towel across their hips would have helped. There'd be no embarrassment for the girl I was with and no need for drawn curtains either. The other girls would see and relax when their turn came. A dreadful procedure would become easy.

I hope you see the pattern. Obsessed with control, our teen boys observed nothing, learned nothing, and risked nothing. That left them withdrawn and miserable. Our teen girls observed, learned to trust, and lightened up. That left them far more comfortable. The guys clearly needed to learn from the girls. Hospital staff can learn from them too.

What about those gown changes? Always done behind closed curtains, no girl contemplating one had seen how I'd handled another girl. Yet that worked because, having decided to trust me, they were willing to take *some* chances. When you trust someone, learning you can trust them more is reassuring, hence those smiles. Also, with those gown changes, I was fully accountable. They were looking up at me. If I'd peeked, even for a second, they would have known. That matters too.

Tired of the European winter, in early December I flew from Athens to Tel Avi. I'd wait out the winter working on a kibbutz and resume my travels as summer approached. Later, a stay in Jerusalem would offer an opportunity to work on an archaeological dig just outside the Old City of Jerusalem.

17. MR. A'S HOSTEL

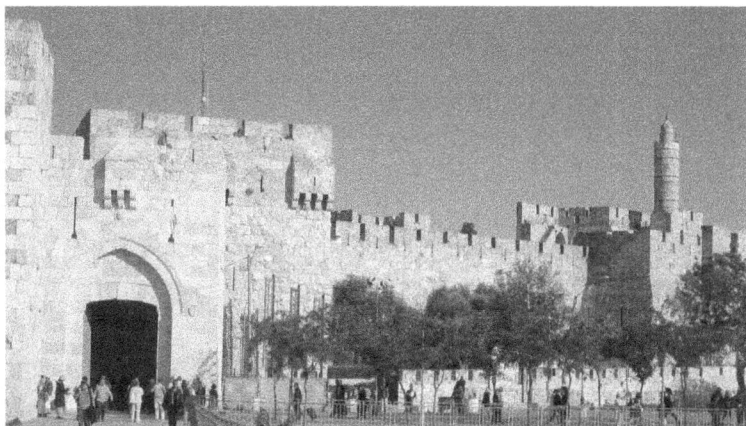

Budget travelers love to share tips about inexpensive places to stay. During my travels, one of the best was a private hostel in the Old City of Jerusalem that cost but a dollar a night. You entered by the Jaffa Gate, pictured above, went up an alley to your left, and the door was about 150 feet in on your right.

Mr. A's, as it was called, was the most fascinating place I'd stay in travels that included a sailing vessel in Stockholm Harbor, a pasture outside Shakespeare's home town, and a castle in Bavaria. What made it unique was the congenial, cooperative atmosphere. I would experience nothing like it elsewhere. For the readers of this book, it offers a chance to move beyond sick teens at a children's hospital and look at healthy young adults from around the world.

Built of stone with arched ceilings and centuries old, Mr. A's resembled the Cairo home of Sallah, played by John Rhys-Davies in *The Raiders of the Lost Ark*. No larger than a modest American home, the living was intimate. Some forty of us, both men and women, shared a single shower and a single toilet. We socialized in a small kitchen or a central courtyard open to the skies. In the Old City, homes resemble fortresses, so we were surrounded by thick stone walls topped by barbed wire and protected by a steel door. That gave a sense of security in a dangerous city.

Veteran travelers all, we were well-behaved. The owner ensured that by renting only to foreigners. Four rooms crowded with narrow beds surrounded the courtyard. Since there was no heating or cooling, they were open to the weather, winter and summer. The largest was for guys, the two smallest were for girls, and a mid-sized one was co-ed, with its guy-to-girl ratio constantly changing. The last was where I stayed. One night the bed next to mine might have an Australian guy in desperate need of a bath. The next it might have a pretty German girl.

How did those girls feel surrounded by so many guys? They loved it, staying night after night and recommending it to other girls. This wasn't a crowded Spanish train filled with creeps shoving and groping. This was like Miss Spain napping next to me. We made them feel comfortable. When Miss Europe wanted a companion for that concert, she need only look around.

Earlier, I hinted that my traveling companionship wasn't unique, that it was being repeated across Europe. Mr. A's concentrated that into one location. Some of the guests were guy/girl pairs with no romantic attachment. I overheard one girl remark to another that she'd been traveling with her guy for two months, and yet he'd made no sexual moves.

These were brave, capable young women, mostly in their twenties, adventurous travelers visiting cultures where the seamier side made life difficult for them. They were curious, wanting to experience the world more vividly than most tourists. Unfortunately, as women that created endless woes. They talked among themselves about those troubles and about the wonderful guys who helped them cope. Out there, they sensed danger. Inside Mr. A's, they were safe. Those guys, recognizing these girls as fellow adventurers unfairly treated because of their sex, were why.

I saw that one night. The hostel's owner was inflexible about his 10 p.m. curfew. When the time came, the steel door at the entrance was bolted shut. No one could enter after that. One night a girl arrived a few minutes late. Finding herself locked out and in a narrow and dark alley, she panicked, pounding on the door and screaming in fear. She wasn't in real danger. There was a police station only a couple of hundred yards away. But she didn't know that and, because she'd been drinking, felt vulnerable.

The owner wouldn't relent, so two guys came to her rescue. He would let guests leave after curfew, so one went out to keep her company. The other waited long enough for the owner to fall asleep and then opened the door for the two. That illustrates why girls loved Mr. A's. They were with guys who appreciated their troubles and were eager to help.

In this book I've contrasted our hospital's teen boys and girls. The boys, it seemed, would allow no exposure, not even of their undies. I could only shake my head. Most nurses had husbands who were far better looking. Many assistants had raised boys. I concluded that for these boys trust mattered little. They wanted to prevent any exposure no matter what. Only control counted. That's why, contrary to what I first thought, my presence made little difference.

Would you be surprised if I told you that the guys with me in that co-ed room at Mr. A's behaved much the same? They did, including me. Like those hospital rooms, Jerusalem gets hot in the summer, and our hostel was no exception. No one wanted to sleep fully clothed. Jeans in particular, needed to come off. Making matters more difficult, there were always lines for the shower and toilet, so changing there meant a wait.

So what's a typical guy to do in a room that has so many girls? His answer was simple. He wore no undies. In their place, he substituted athletic shorts. I only saw one exception, a guy who didn't get the 'men must wear athletic shorts while traveling' memo. Mr. Brief was wearing white cotton briefs. The other guys hounded him so mercilessly, he left after but one night.

I understood their thinking, because I was doing the same. I traveled with three dark athletic shorts, easily washed and dried, so I'd be ready for any situation. Taking off pants was no more embarrassing than leaving them on. That's very masculine. A guy wants to be in control, so he can deal with any eventuality. Having underclothes that were outer clothes solved the undressing issue.

Would athletic shorts ease the unhappiness I saw with our teen boys? Certainly, the only underclothing that Teens offered those boys were those dread white cotton briefs. Forced to wear them, our boys felt they had to stay covered up, however miserable that made them. Supplying shorts would have also made our clothing inventory simpler. Three or four sizes could handle both boys and girls.

How about the girls who so generously shared that co-ed room at Mr. A's with us? How did they deal with that heat and the need to remove jeans or skirts? First, I should offer a disclaimer. Like the other guys, I would look away when they undressed. That seemed polite. But in the end that mattered little. As with those post-op girls, I couldn't just look at my feet. We all knew—both boys and girls—what the other was wearing to stay cool overnight.

The girls could not have been more different. Indeed, from my masculine perspective I can only conclude that women view clothing quite differently from men. Underneath their jeans or skirts, they wore undies, almost always white and most so brief they barely covered. A t-shirt or blouse on top resulted in the skimpiest of mini-skirts. As a guy, that struck me as impractical. Traveling on a budget meant that every few days these girls had to scrub those underthings by hand to keep them white. Yet, to my knowledge no girl ever suggested to her peers that should change. When it came to clothing, the two sexes were certainly different.

Like the boys, there was one exception, a girl who was placed in the bed next to mine. Another girl and savvy traveler made fun of this girl's doctrinaire feminism, telling her. "Why do I need feminism? I've always been able to do anything I wanted." In her own way, Miss Tea was as clueless as Mr. Brief. She was attending the first college in the U.S. to go co-ed, and yet she didn't know what to do in this most co-ed of hostels. Most girls I met traveling had a sensible skirt. Reaching below their knees, it was comfortable, easily cared for, and perfect for when jeans were too casual. Miss Tea's dress was nothing like that. It was what a woman might have worn to a ladies tea party in the 1950s. Not practical, it needed constant attention, frequent ironing, and probably required a slip underneath.

I'm not sure what Miss Tea made of me in a bed only a foot from hers. I did my best to appear harmless, but I can't recall a word that passed between us. I and the other guys were too much for her. At lights out, as she lay down on her bed in her tea dress, I thought that surely she wouldn't wear that all night. Sometime later, when there were no more lines for the shower or toilet, she'll slip off and change to something practical. She'd didn't. When I woke the next morning, she was still in that tea party dress. Like Mr. Brief, she didn't return for another night.

So yes, while I'm describing boys and girls in generalities, there are exceptions that support the generalities. In a sense, both Mr. Brief and Miss Tea had flipped their sex's distinctive behaviors. Mr. Brief gave up control to have underwear that was distinctively masculine. Miss Tea wore her feminine clothing on the outside, where it couldn't help but draw unwanted attention from creepy guys.

Having covered the exceptions, we'll now see if these traveling young women can help us understand the teen girls I would later care for. Keep in mind that, while I could easily understand traveling young men, since I was one, I can only guess about their female counterparts. Feel free to follow your own interpretation.

First, why was there this great distinction in what was worn underneath? To understand, recall that men and women dress differently to highlight their masculinity or femininity. For men on the road that was easy. We liked grunge, so traveling was great fun. For women traveling rough, it wasn't. Their clothing needed to deter creeps. Showers might be days apart. Makeup was impossible in the heat. As guys who'd grown tired of dusty streets and crowded buses, we found them pretty, but I suspect they didn't feel that way. Their out-of-sight underwear was the only way they could express their femininity. It told them, "Yes, I'm still a woman." The more feminine it was, the better—hence tiny, white, and certainly nothing like a man's dark athletic shorts. The girls on Teens often did the same, preferring what they brought from home, also typically tiny and white, to the baggy undies the hospital provided.

The second issue arose when these girls found themselves in co-ed housing at Mr. A's. What were they to do? There was an option. Most had ordinary shorts as well as jeans. They could wait in line for the toilet or shower and change there. I assure you, I wasn't making a study, but I can't recall that happening. Some changed as soon was we moved indoors after that unlit courtyard grew too dark for socializing. Most, a bit more modest, changed just before or after lights out a little after ten. That's the same casual versus careful distinction I saw with the girls on Teens.

There was another similarity. When I first worked with post-op girls, I expected them to wear more when I became their caregiver. To my surprise, that didn't happen. On a Monday, when I started with them, I might have three girls with nothing underneath and one with undies. Seven days later, there'd be the same three-to-one ratio. When they decided I could be trusted, there was no halfway—they really trusted. I was amazed, but they saw that as natural.

Mr. A's was similar, but with some five guys in the room rather than just me. The girls looked around, concluded they could trust us, and felt they would be insulting us to act otherwise. Off came their jeans or skirts, so they could sleep cool. How they acted afterward also mattered. Cowering beneath sheets would have said, "Don't look at me. I don't trust you." Prancing about the room that lightly dressed would have said the exact opposite. They did neither. They undressed and sat demurely on their beds until lights out.

The third issue was these girls ready acceptance of us. Recall what Miss Naples told me about her irritation when those creepy Italian males "accidentally" bumped up against her. She was picking up on their intentions and furious about what that meant. Not sensing any malicious intent, the girls at Mr. A's relaxed.

I saw that one afternoon when I returned to Mr. A's and immediately headed for the shower. It was entered though a door and about four or five steps up. At the top and to the left was a tiny room that was the shower—no curtains, just the shower. Starting up, I saw a woman's underwear hanging from a hook. The room was obviously occupied. I turned around and called up that I would watch the door while she came down and locked it, which she did as quiet as a mouse. Yes, she should have been more careful, but not locking that door did hint at how safe she felt at Mr. A's.

Why was there this striking male-female distinction at the hostel and at the hospital, with guys obsessing over the control and girls relying on trust? The answer lies in the differing circumstances each experiences when troubles arise.

A man typically see himself in a dangerous world against which he must pit his abilities. To remain safe, he must manage events in his favor. That's why control matters so much. If he loses control, disaster may follow. That's also why his response typically involves fight or flight. Fight when you can win and flee when you cannot. That requires being free to choose one or the other. Finally, it's why he respects guys he can depend on in a pinch, such as my Mr. Big, and loathes cowards such as Mr. Chicken.

On the other hand, while a girl will sense those same dangers and may even feel them more strongly, her typically smaller size and physical strength means she instinctively seeks someone stronger to handle fight-or-fight situations. Since a Miss Athletic is rare, that usually means a man, but not just any man. He must be one she can trust. A man who can't be trusted is worse than useless. You might put it this way. When a man faces danger, he asks if another man will fight *alongside* him. When a woman faces danger, she asks if that man will fight *for* her. That's why she is drawn to responses that will increase a man's commitment to her—tending and befriending.

Tending means offering help and hoping assistance will be given in return. That was why, when those girls in Brindisi approached me, they offered to share their lunch. By tending, a woman is saying, "See I'm helping you, so please help me." On Teens, some girls did that, catering beautifully to my emotional needs. Often, they weren't the main beneficiaries. Instead, the encouragement they offered gave me the strength to defy an often-cruel system, as I'll explain in a couple of chapters when I discuss Dan and Pala.

Just as fleeing is the opposite of fighting, so *befriending* is the opposite of tending. Instead of saying, "I can help you," it says "I need your help." A woman does that by heightening her vulnerability. On a date, her clothing and high heels make her *less* able to defend herself and thus *more* dependent on the guy she's with. She needs him more, in the hope that he'll do more. That was true traveling. Miss Spain napped next to me like a little kitten. Miss Naples didn't mind being bumped. The girls at Mr. A's slept next to us. That same befriending happened on Teens. While teen boys were infuriated by their helplessness, many teen girls saw it as a way to win my assistance.

Those differences make sense. While taking Miss Europe to that concert, suppose I saw someone dangerous ahead. That's not hypo-

thetical. As I write, Jerusalem is troubled by knife-bearing terrorists. One recent attack was but a few hundred yards from Mr. A's
former location. A killer with a knife is difficult to handle. To do
that I *must* control events. I need to *know* that, if I turn aside, Miss
Europe will follow. I also need to be sure that, if a terrorist pulls a
knife, she will move behind me. That makes defending her easier.
Finally, if matters turn still worse, I need to be certain that, if I say
"Run," she'll flee while I delay the attacker. That's why her trust and
cooperation matters. It makes what I must do easier.

The opposite can be dreadful. Years ago, I went walking late at
night in a wooded area of a major city with a friend. Every time
the bushes closed in, I thought "mugger." I was unhappy to see her
dart ahead, as if eager to meet such a person. I made a mental note
to never take her to any place dangerous again. Yes, it's male ego,
but it also makes sense. As men, we like to *feel* in control because
we often *need* to be in control. Bad things happen when we aren't.
How does that apply to hospitals? Hospitals can be as stressful as a
city haunted by terrorists or muggers. Men who're genuinely masculine get upset when they lose control. Hospitals should give them as
much control as possible. That's where we failed.

Miss Europe proved a much better companion. Lacking Miss
Athletic's strong physique, she knew walking alone to that concert
posed serious risks. She not only wasn't powerful enough to handle a
knife-bearing terrorist, her weakness might attract an attacker who
would let the two of us pass unmolested. That's why she wanted me
along. And that's why I enjoyed taking her.

Nor did the mere presence of a man guarantee her safety. All
men are not equal. Going with a creep or with Mr. Chicken would
have made her situation worse. She needed a guy she could depend
on. To achieve that, she distinguished good guys from bad, took
advantage of tend and befriend to attract a good one, and cooperated with him. She was smart.

We turn now to the downside of this marvelous feminine ability
to trust so completely. What if a woman's trust proves unjustified?
What if a guy she thought good proves to be a creep? That's next,
and it is *very* relevant to hospitals.

18. Infuriated Girls

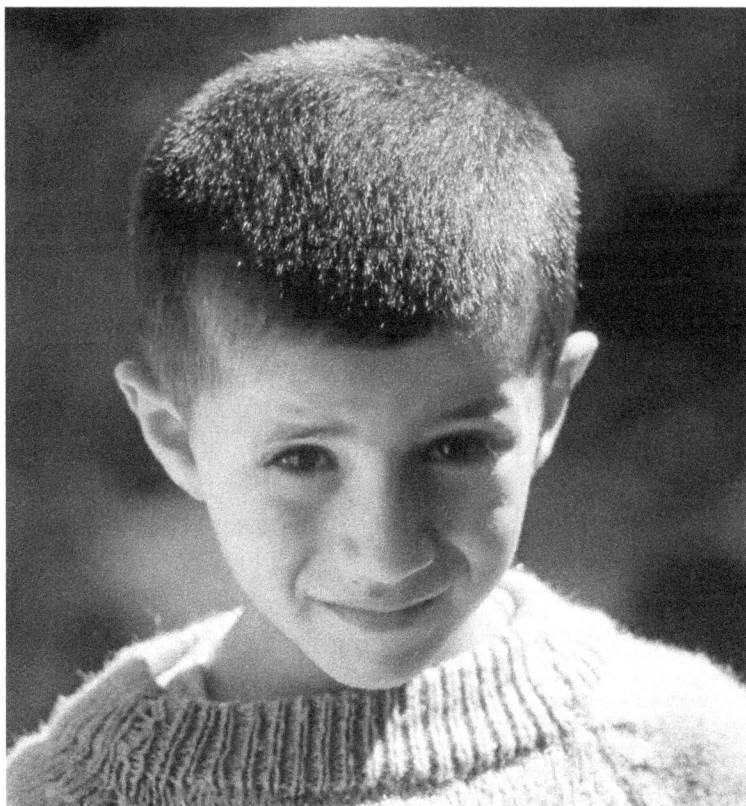

Before I met Miss Spain, I briefly visited Morocco. There I met a guy who'd just had a terrifying experience. Intending to buy illicit drugs, he'd gone with two men to a shack on the outskirts of Fez. They proved more interested in extortion than dealing. If he didn't give them his money, he was warned, they'd kill and bury him in the sand dunes of the Sahara.

Displaying remarkable calm, he told them that he only had enough for the ferry back to Spain, where he'd left the rest of his money. Underneath the table, however, he was slipping bills out of his wallet into a sock, all but for one, which he hoped was for $20. He got lucky, because it was. To me, he readily admitted he never should have trusted those drug dealers.

Trusting is one of the most important decisions we make in life and being trusted is one of the greatest compliments we can receive. I adored those post-op girls for trusting me despite my clumsiness. They made what would have otherwise been a difficult job much easier. The same was true of Miss Spain, Miss Naples, Miss Delicate, Miss Europe, and all the other girls I met traveling. Riding the rails of Europe and later staying at Mr. A's would have been far less interesting without them. But their ready trust, which so amazed me, had a serious downside. Those young women could be hurt badly if their trust was violated. That's what this chapter is about. Given the importance of a patient's trust in caregivers, it's an area that medicine and nursing need to explore more deeply.

I saw violations of trust while staying in Jerusalem. The archaeological dig where I was volunteering ended work at lunch, so I'd head back to Mr. A's in early afternoon. I would shower and recuperate from a morning spent on an east-facing slope under the blazing Middle-Eastern sun. The solar-powered shower only had enough hot water for a few showers, so I did my best to be early.

As I rested through the afternoon, other guests arrived. The women were often upset and looking for a guy to talk with, sometimes picking me. I knew what had them upset, one or more Arabs males (not men) they'd encountered that day. Fortunately, I had the sense not to make the Typical Male Mistake of telling them the Practical Thing To Do. That was to forget that 'learning about other cultures' nonsense and treat those creeps with the contempt they deserved. I didn't need to say that, because they'd already learned.

I should add that all Arabs need not be avoided. Arab women, while they didn't go out of their way to talk to foreigners, were pleasant. Arab kids were great and would surround me when I hiked into a West Bank village. This chapter starts with a picture of one who came up to me at Herod's Gate and, through his grandfather, asked me to take his picture.

I often rode Arab buses, and I remember a crowded one in particular. Every time a woman would board the bus, whether she was young or old, one of the young boys would get up and offer her his seat. They were still under the influence of mothers and grandmothers. Older men in shops could be pushy, but I kept in mind that what they sold that day was probably all the money they had to feed their family that night. That's why I felt bad bargaining aggressively over prices.

That aside, young Arab males were vile. As a guy, I could cope with their obvious lies. They just wanted my money. Women had to deal with other vices. And yes, I admit that there was a selection bias at play. Creepy Arab males targeted foreign women, particularly those alone, while the ones who weren't creepy did nothing and thus weren't counted. But to justify that excuse you must explain why the latter did nothing about the creeps. In the end, everyone in a group bears some responsibility for those in it who behave badly.

Some afternoons I'd have a different conversation. On those days, a girl would excitedly tell me about a young Arab male she'd met that day, and how she was looking forward to a date that evening. He was so nice, she said, and seemed to like her.

"Bosh," I thought, as a well-seasoned traveler. In my travels I'd only met one I'd trust, a medical student whose Hebron home I visited. I'd been stuck by his honesty. For the rest, distrust made more sense. These young Arabs differed in two ways from their Southern European counterparts. First, rather than anonymously bump or grope, they'd start with charm and compliments, only later showing their true colors. Second, their policy of deception meant they typically approached a woman alone. Their fake charm worked poorly with two women. The one not being targeted saw through their lies. That may explain why, unlike Southern Europe, I can't recall a situation in Israel where I had to reassure women who were traveling together. They found safety in numbers.

Alas, I knew those girls weren't ready for bluntness, so I waited for them to return that evening. Every time, the girl came back infuriated. This guy, seemingly interested in her, proved only interested in sex. I couldn't tell her, "I told you so," because I hadn't. But I could listen, calm her down and help her with what she wanted most, which was not to generalize from one creep to all men. Those women were showing good sense. Recall that old adage that when you're thrown from a horse, quickly get back on so you don't acquire a lifelong fear of horses. If you're a woman who gets mistreated by a creep, spend time with good men as a corrective.

There was another situation at Mr. A's worthy of comment. To expand on my experience on the dig, in the evening I often read a book about a famous archaeological dig in nearby Jericho. Some evenings, the ratio in the co-ed room tilted heavily female. When that happened, I'd pretend to read, but actually listen to my roommates talk about their experiences, good and bad, with men met while traveling. I didn't consciously draw on those experiences when I began to work on Teens, but I'm sure they helped.

How important is it for anyone who is subject to sexual harassment to deal quickly with bad situations such as these—including those in hospitals? Critically important. About a decade after I worked on Teens I had an experience which illustrates that. What happened is complicated, so I'll just describe what matters here.

At a church I was attending, I met a charming Asian girl we'll call Miss Cute, because she was. On our first meeting, she volunteered her phone number and then proceeded, time and again, to say no when I asked her out—but always sweetly. She was testing me much like those girls I had met traveling. After about six weeks, as I grew weary of being turned down, she suggested a bike ride. All seemed well for about two weeks after that.

Then Miss Cute turned into a forbidding stone wall. She wouldn't talk with or even look at me. All my efforts to discover what I'd done wrong came to naught. After about a month, I was ready to give up, but decided to do her a small favor. With that, something clicked, and she opened up. She told me she was so upset about a guy that she was getting only three to four hours sleep a night. That meant the problem was a Mr. Scum rather than me. A hypothetical situation she later mentioned suggested an attempted date rape. Since she was tiny, that must have been terrifying.

Miss Cute had done the opposite of what those girls at Mr. A's did when they sought out good guys to vent their frustrations. Badly hurt, she had excluded all men from her life until, in desperation, she turned to me. She unbolted the door, yanked me inside, and then bolted it shut again, still not having anything to do with other men. At first I didn't realize what I was in for.

The chief difficulty was that Miss Cute was exceptionally kind, all tend and befriend with no fight or flight. She could not settle her troubled feelings by simply loathing Mr. Scum, as much as he deserved it. That disappointed me. I visualized being with her when he appeared. I was wearing the boots I wore mountain climbing—thick, heavily padded, and with a long steel shank. I'd kick Mr. Scum in the shins, then stomp on his feet to inflict considerable pain. Alas, at that point my imagination failed to keep up with my desires. Before I could give him a well-deserved kick in the groin, he fled, absolutely terrified. That would have felt good.

Events took a different path. You may have heard of *cognitive dissonance*, which is the discomfort that results from conflicting experiences and beliefs. That's what Miss Cute and I went through. One moment, I was the only guy she trusted. The next, I was "Mike the Date Rapist." That drove me nuts, but showed what she was going through, bouncing wildly from one extreme to another. For six months that went on, until she again slept normally. Alas, our relationship didn't survive the transition. She wanted a close friendship. Exhausted, I couldn't endure anything that wasn't casual, so we drifted apart.

What can be learned from these girls about in-hospital accusations of sexual harassment? First, that situations ranging from merely embarrassing to allegations of actual sexual assault *must be dealt with quickly and effectively*. Don't allow negative feelings to fester and turn sour.

In all too many hospitals, the first reaction is to call a lawyer who makes matters worse, typically suggesting that the hospital admit to nothing, not even the most obvious of facts. Faced with complaints from patients or reports from nurses, hospitals go into Three Monkeys Mode. They hear no evil, see no evil and speak no evil. Of course, that only applies to themselves. Defending themselves, they implicitly criticize nurses or patients who've made charges. That makes matters worse. Much of the time, those who've been hurt simply want an apology and an assurance it won't happen again. Deprived of that, they may go to the media or hire a lawyer. A small problem becomes costly.

As I write this, the very hospital where I worked is facing a lawsuit by a young woman who was a patient in the locked psychiatric unit. She claims that it failed protect her from a male patient with a history of sexual assault. In the past, hospitals have usually won in court because the situation typically degenerated into 'he said, she said,' with he winning by default. That's changing. In an age of smartphones, the person making charges may have a recording that backs up her claims. Then hospitals will pay.

Second, while the situations I've described involve women discussing their frustrations about men, we should never forget that they were *choosing* the men they talked with. They think, "I trust him. If I talk with him, he'll listen, and I'll feel better." That may not work in a hospital where all is formal and impersonal. Strangers from an "Incident Quick Response Team" may do more harm than good. Consider sending someone of the same sex with a caring, helping personality.

Third, talk should *always* result in concrete action. I saw that traveling. The girls who paired with me received immediate relief. As soon as I appeared, those creeps vanished. Patients should be just as quickly and surely comforted. The person accused should no longer be in a position to upset the patient. For that to happen, those involved must have the authority to act. They can't just say, "I'll see what I can do." They should have the authority to do.

Fourth, not all issues will center on what men do to women. Even when a man is the chief offender, a woman patient may be more upset at being betrayed by staff women she though she could trust than at the creep himself. Don't assume anything. Always listen to what patients are saying.

Finally, a hospital keep from being overwhelmed by allegations by creating a all-around healthy climate in which even small problems become rare. That'll make the more serious problems even rarer.

In the next chapter, we'll look at how a hospital can fail in small ways that might, in certain circumstances, lead to more serious allegations of wrong-doing. And yes, we're back to those hated linen changes again.

19. Overwhelmed Pala

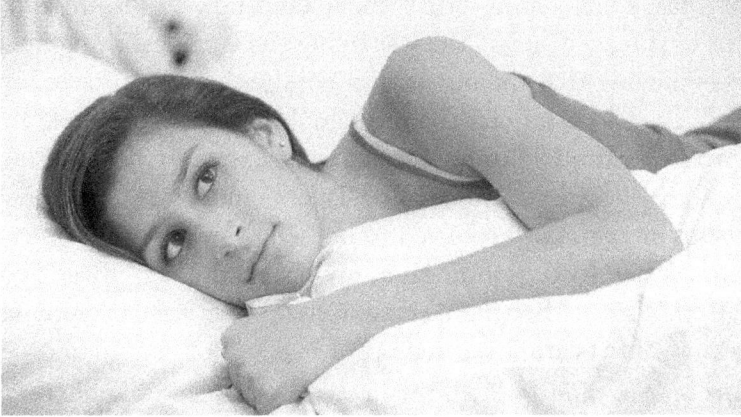

Early one Thursday afternoon, I admitted Dan, a brown-haired boy of about twelve. He was accompanied by his parents, who'd been told the boy had leukemia. Normally, we hit the ground running, but not this time. None of our specialists came. Only a resident dropped in, and he only to apologize for the delay, citing a medical conference going on.

The next morning, I grew ticked off as I saw the parents waiting by their son's bed, worry on their faces. From long experience, I knew what Dan's treatment would feel like and considered talking with them about that. But I could see my limitations. The tests that would more precisely diagnosis his leukemia hadn't been run, so no one knew much about the challenges he faced. Beside, our specialists would be most unhappy to discover that a mere assistant had given medical advice.

So I hit on a better idea. We had movies-on-demand, and Dan was one of the lucky few with a working television. I brought him a notebook listing what films were available and suggested *The Wizard of Oz*. Our patients liked what it said about facing fears. I liked it because, as I told one boy, a song reminded me of someone.

Ding dong! The witch is dead.
Which old witch? The wicked witch.
Ding dong! The wicked witch is dead.

I had good reason for feeling that way. The substitute head nurse, who'd kindly overlooked my Great Linen Rebellion, was back caring for patients. The returning head nurse was not winning our hearts. Ms. Ding Dong didn't understand how to inspire and had turned to threats instead. She was doing the stupidest thing imaginable—believing that the nurses at a children's hospital were unmotivated. They were among the most highly motivated people I have ever worked with. Claiming Teens had become rotten while she was away, she attacked us, threatening layoffs and firings. She tried to get me to inform, but I resolved to not let a word of criticism escape my lips. When I left months later, my resignation letter was a barely veiled criticism of her management style. She wasn't happy about that, but I didn't care. I was fed up.

A couple of months later, the hospital's chaplain told me that just after I'd left, there'd been a mass exodus of nurses. Almost a quarter of them resigned in only a few weeks. At first, I was confused. I could see why those nurses *ought* to be unhappy, but I'd heard no one complain. Then I realized that, when people are merely a little unhappy, they complain. When they're extremely unhappy, they say nothing, find another job, and quit with short notice. The spring timing of their departure may have been to get jobs before newly graduating nurses entered the market.

Now back to Dan. I understood how hard it was for his parents to complain. They were desperate to get good care and didn't want to make trouble. My attempts to ease their anxiety did not pass unnoticed by Ms. Ding Dong, who called me in for a talk. As far as I knew, she never praised our hard-working nurses or assistants. She certainly never had a good word for me. Now I had to face her wrath. She was unhappy with what I'd done. She claimed that I should not have "wasted time" explaining those movies. Instead, I should have been changing bed linens, generating numbers for her superiors. Yes, bed linens, the bane of my existence. I was glad she hadn't been around earlier. My Great Linen Rebellion would have become a Battle Royale. We would have fought to the death.

I said nothing, but wasn't repentant. Sixteen months with kids who had leukemia made them special. I hated seeing Dan neglected.

If that happened again, I would have done exactly the same. Stubbornness can be a virtue.

A month or so later, a girl I'll call Pala put me a similar situation. She was a slender fourteen-year-old. Like Dan, she had been newly diagnosed with leukemia, although her treatment was moving with the usual bewildering speed. On the afternoon of her second day, my nurse asked me to assist a resident with her spinal tap. That would reveal if her leukemic cells had crossed into her spinal fluid.

Unfortunately, this resident was incompetent, inserting a needle into the small of her back three times without getting a drop of fluid. He stalked off without a word, leaving me with a distraught girl. When I cleaned up afterward, I discovered why he'd failed. The spinal tap kit he used was clearly marked for infants only. The needle was too short. He hadn't learn Rule One of Medicine—check and recheck everything. Then check again.

Alone in the exam room with Pala, I faced a problem. I could smell urine. This frightened little Munchkin had been so traumatized, she'd wet herself. She shared a room with three other girls, so I knew she didn't want to go back smelling like that. But helping her put me in a bind. The day had been rough. I was far behind before I'd been asked to assist with that spinal tap. The resident's blunders had put me twenty more minutes behind. Evening shift might complain, and I'd face another session with Ms. Ding Dong—not a pleasant thought.

I had a choice. Working with younger children had made me an expert on wet clothes. Hospitalized, they often forgot their potty training. Changing was easy. I'd stand them beside the bed, slip off their wet clothes, put on new ones, and then sit them in a chair while I changed their sheets. I did that often enough, I was quick. The faster I was, the sooner they could go back to sleep. In a hospital, sleep is a great blessing.

I could do the same with Pala, but for one hitch. She was fourteen rather than four. Even though Ms. Ding Dong did not care, that mattered. Pala was in shock from all she'd been through and wouldn't protest. But that wasn't the point. What mattered was what I *should* do not what I *could* do. I had an alternative. I could turn around while she changed herself, slow though that might be.

Ms. Ding Dong would not be happy about that, since I could have used that time to change those infernal sheets.

Needing time to think, I asked Pala to remain lying down until I returned with clean clothes. Keep in mind the broader context. When I first began working with children who had leukemia, I had to cope with inflicting pain. I hated that and resolved that, if I could ease their suffering in the slightest, I would. What I could do was pitifully small.

Pala's situation was similar, but with embarrassment rather than pain. She'd been going through hell. In the past two days, her world had collapsed. The day before, she'd been told that she had a disease that could kill her in mere months. Today meant brutally invasive tests, including a bone marrow aspiration. Tomorrow, she'd begin her chemotherapy, followed by a grim aftermath that would last for weeks. Her hair would fall out, and she'd grow weak. She'd hear no good news for six months, after which she might be told that she remained in remission, but must wait for years to find out if she'd been cured. Still later, she'd have to worry about the long-term consequences of her chemotherapy. Not embarrassing her now might not be much, but it was all I could do. I couldn't wave my arms and send her home cured.

As I returned to the exam room, I resolved to take the gentle approach, come what may. When I saw Pala curled up, so terrified and desperately alone, I knew that was right. To ease what she was going through, I'd take on every cold-hearted Ms. Ding Dong in existence—and enjoy it. I also made a mental note to send every patient about to get a spinal tap to the toilet beforehand, so no one else would face this problem again.

I faced away while Pala changed and all ended well. Evening shift was in a good mood. No one complained about work left undone. Fortunately, Ms. Ding Dong wasn't omniscient. She huddled in her office, rarely mixing with staff. What she did not hear about, she couldn't attack. I'd defied the nit-pickers obsessed with metrics, treated a frightened girl kindly, and gotten away with it. Yeah!

Well, maybe. Long-term, I faced a problem. As I walked Pala back to her bed, two feelings—a hope and a fear—passed through my mind. I hoped that, just before she went to sleep that night, she'd feel good about a clothing change done right. That wasn't much, but it was a tiny light in her dark world.

The fear would haunt me during my last months at the hospital. The cooperative relationships I'd established with these girls had a serious flaw. It was no longer about my winning their trust. They trusted me so consistently, I no longer worried about that. Nor was it better techniques. By the end of that summer, what I was doing was almost as good as could be done. It was simply that I was a guy and some girls valued their modesty enough to need ways to opt out of me. That I understood and respected.

In practice, not choosing me meant choosing their nurse. That's where a key difference between Hem-Onc and Teens mattered. On Hem-Onc nights, we paid little attention to distinctions between nurse and assistant. When a nurse took her half-hour break just after her 4 a.m. medications, I became Hem-Onc's nurse, flipping a patient's IV from medication-dispensing to maintenance and whatever else was required. I did that hundreds of times and never made a mistake. In exchange, when a frightened child needed rocking to sleep, for the time that took—typically 45 minutes—the nurse did my work. Sharing worked well.

Unfortunately, little sharing was allowed on Teens, and most of the burden fell on our nurses. They had to do some of my work, but it was almost impossible for me to return the favor. Two bed-bound girls might be next to one another. One regularly asked me for a bedpan. The other never did. Did the second have an unusually large bladder? No, she was merely waiting until her nurse came around. Yet if one of those girls' IV beeped, I could not help, no matter how trivial the fix. That was the problem.

The nurses I worked with were marvelous. They never complained or lectured these girls on how busy they were. For all their casualness about undress, they never told those girls to quit being hung up on modesty and call on me instead of them. They were kind. They were rebelling against the folly of the "staff are not male or female" as much as I was.

In fact, there was one area where our nurses concluded that their medical orders were humiliating and refused to do them.

That involved girls with anorexia nervosa. During my ten months, I cared for three girls with it. None were in immediate danger. One even became so fed up, she dressed in street clothes, walked out, and found her way home thirty miles away. No, we were simply giving them a place to stay while they were counseled. The first time I cared for one, the nurse told me there were two rules. First, we should never talk to them about food. Second, they could not get up and use the toilet. They must endure bedpans.

The first rule was obeyed without exception, and for that I was glad. The only conversation I wanted to have about food came when I brought them lunch. Looking down at a tray that held no more than skim milk and a green salad without dressing. I wanted to scream, "Eat, you've got to eat!" I'm sure their psychiatrist would not have regarded that as helpful.

The second rule was ignored or, to be more specific, deliberately rendered ineffective. Our nurses saw that no-toilet rule as demeaning. To enforce it, as staff we needed to put up the side rails on their beds. That we never did. Noticing that, these girls slipped out of bed and used the toilet when we weren't around. Neither we nor those girls told their psychiatrist about that little game. And no, the reason for that rule wasn't to make sure these girls didn't vomit up what little they were eating (bulimia). That could have been handled by having us stand outside the toilet. The rule was simply mean, and we refused to be mean.

Bedpans for other patients were handled with equal kindness. Hospital policy dictated that, as the assistant, I should handle them all. Instead, there was an unwritten rule. If a girl asked a nurse, the nurse took care of it. There were no Maria-like "Mike will take care of that" referrals. For that, I was glad. Perhaps once or twice a day a girl would ask me to get her nurse without explaining why. I didn't ask, since I knew the reason. The nurses, wonderful as they were, fit that into their overloaded schedules.

Ah, but playing fast and loose with the rules came with a risk. I feared Ms. Ding Dong would use some incident—such as Pala's clothing change—to dictate that, as the assistant, I must handle *all* the embarrassing work. Our nurses would still cheat, bless their hearts, but defying Ms. Ding Dong's dictate would make life harder for everyone. That worried me, so I did my best to keep that vile idea from reaching her troll's cave at our entrance.

Fortunately, that never happened, so I need not explain more. Administrative meanness was plentiful and growing steadily worse, often targeting the best nurses. But it never focused on embarrassment. It was obsessed with metrics and mistakes. Harsh criticism led to that mass exodus mere weeks after my resignation. Those who want to know more can read *Senior Nurse Mentor*, where I describe the problems and offer practical solutions. That book is also great for students needing to acquire a feel for hospital politics before facing its horrors for real. Forewarned is forearmed.

Having praised the helpfulness of our nurses, I should also praise some marvelously helpful patients. I hated all the busy work of day shift, but when morale plummeted after Ms. Ding Dong returned, I became discouraged. I shouldn't have to fight to treat my patients kindly, I thought, particularly those with a disease that could kill, such as leukemia. I could have become depressed and given up.

Enter several teen girls, typically those in for long stays. Sensing my discouragement, they went out of their way to cheer me up. Even when I wasn't assigned to their cluster, they would look for me. That was a marvelous example of tend and befriend, with me being the one tended. Even more amazing, their maladies were far worse than anything I faced.

At sixteen, Grace had just been diagnosed with systematic lupus erythematosus (SLE), one of the auto-immune diseases I hate. A picture I have of her shows the characteristic butterfly-shaped flushing of SLE on her face. In for lab tests, she could go where she wanted, so she'd accompany me when I was with other girls. Always cheerful, she helped me endure the grind.

Another girl was even more heart-breaking. A few years earlier, Nancy had been diagnosed with abdominal cancer. To treat it, she'd received radiation. Given only on one side of her body, the muscles on that side atrophied, causing her spine to twist. She could have had the same spinal fusion we gave to other girls, but elected not, given that her cancer seemed certain to kill her. She defeated the cancer, but too late for back surgery. Her spine was now so distorted, she could not stand. Yet despite that, she'd dress herself, hop into a wheelchair and come looking for me with her beautiful smile. I was most flattered.

Grace and Nancy illustrate why I don't understand hospital staff who dislike patients. Patients were the best part of my work. Those who went out of their way to be cheer me up also gave me the emotional strength to care for other patients too overwhelmed to charm me, such as Pala. I could do more, because they strengthened me. Hospitals need to encourage that. Patients should not be treated as passive, incapable of contributing to their care or that of other patients. Allow them to play a role.

In a chapter of *My Nights with Leukemia* called "Hanna the Most Brave," I describe how Hanna, a chatty seventeen-year-old girl, wheelchair bound, befriended Tanya, a shy, twelve-year-old girl dying of a brain tumor with no family present. Hanna did what we as staff lacked the time to do, stay with Tanya and talk with her during her final weeks. She willingly chose to befriend someone she knew was going to die. She is one of the bravest people I've ever known.

Earlier, I wrote about the role that choice played in patient comfort. Being able to accept or reject embarrassing situations made patients feel more in control and thus more cooperative. That takes care of most situations but not all. Pala was an exception to my usual practice of simply letting patients choose to accept or reject embarrassing circumstances. She was so overwhelmed, being shoved from one test to another, that she was in no condition to decide. Instead, I chose for her, picking the least humiliating option. That worked out well and was well worth the two or three minutes it took.

In the next chapter we'll look at situations where neither choice nor embarrassment seem to apply. What should we do in those cases? Should we just assume that embarrassment doesn't exist and do what comes easiest?

20. Helpless Mimi

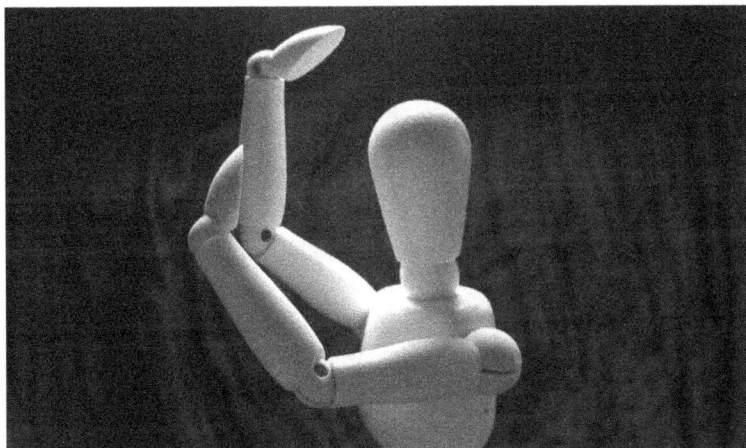

I forget the specifics, but events must have gone like this. While I was at lunch, Don was admitted, probably though our ER, and assigned a bed on C cluster. He was an athletic, twenty-year-old black man in the midst of a serious sickle-cell crisis. For that, he was getting IV fluids and morphine.

Don wasn't our usual cower-beneath-his-sheets guy. In comparison to him, even the post-op girls were overdressed. Some had nothing under their gowns. He did not even have a gown, although I'm not sure why. When he arrived, I suspect he felt so hot and uncomfortable that he refused to wear one. Also, this was summer, so his west-facing room was miserably hot.

His pain and the morphine soon rendered him unconscious. As he thrashed about, he kicked down his sheets. When I checked on him, I replaced them. I also became ticked off at his nurse. He's getting a huge dose of morphine, I told myself, she should check up on him more often.

Yes, I was stupid, incredibly so. I should have realized she wasn't comfortable with going into an unconscious, naked guy almost her age. All I needed to do was flip the circumstances around to see that. I could have made her work easier by putting a gown on him.

But that thought never came to me, because his undress wasn't a issue with me. Stupid!

Later, I'd experience much the same feelings as that nurse, although they would linger for days rather than hours. Mimi was a fourteen-year-old girl who had been admitted with the classic symptoms of one form of catatonia. Her diagnosis seemed straightforward, but for some reason our psychiatrists delayed running a test that would make it definitive. While they dithered, I fretted.

I had reason to fret. When I did my own tests for catatonia, she was a perfect match. When I turned her on her side in an awkward position with one arm elevated, she remained that way, her arm only slowly sinking back down. That's not a coma or drug overdose. That's catatonia. It's like those flexible, wooden statues dancers use to illustrate various poses and is called "waxy flexibility."

Her condition meant she was in no condition to bathe herself. That mattered because day-shift assistants were supposed to see that patients got a bath at least once every three days. The first day passed easily. "Too early for that bath," I could say. On the second day I became worried. Since we didn't know when she'd last bathed, she might already be due for one.

On the morning of her third day, I was most unhappy. Today was the day when it must happen. But as I ran through possible scenarios, I felt uncomfortable. If she's been able to say, "I know the nurse is busy, so it's OK if you do it," I would have been fine. Her choosing would have been like my other patients. But she merely lay there, as oblivious to her surroundings as a dance doll. Even worse, I couldn't come up with a way to give her a sponge bath that seemed different from a molester with a drugged victim.

I went to lunch in a quiet panic. Afternoons were usually slower, which meant my last excuse would vanish. When I came back, I was ecstatic when a fellow assistant told me that she'd given the girl a bath while I was gone. I could have hugged her! That illustrates why I was infuriated at administrative attacks on fellow staff. I worked with good people. I could be depend on them.

Notice that these two incidents differ from those we've discussed thus far. In those earlier situations, despite any pressures that patients might be under, they could say no or at least signal their displeasure. Not so here. Both Don and Mimi were not only unable to say no, the issue was like a question philosophers ask, "If a tree falls in the forest and no one is around, does it make a sound?" In this case, the question is, "if patients are unaware of what happens to them, are they being embarrassed?"

One answer is Tolkien-like, seeing the trees in that wood as Ents who hear the sound of other trees falling and sympathize. In a hospital, those include staff and other patients, who may become upset. Also, comas may not last forever. How a patient feels when looking back counts. That's why it's best to assume that, if embarrassment would exist when the patient was conscious, it exists in some sense when they're unconscious. They still need to be treated with respect.

Here's another example. One afternoon I got a call to transport a fourteen-year-old boy in a coma from Admissions to Teens. "Admissions," I thought as I went to get him, "that is crazy. People in comas come through the ER."

Admissions was right. Jeff had been the victim of an accident in a nearby state two months earlier. A typical teen boy, on family vacation he was having the time of his life jumping sand dunes with a dirt bike, coming down hard and fast. Then he came down too hard and lost control, suffering broken bones and a serious concussion. His bones had healed, but he remained in a coma.

Jeff's family faced a problem. As middle-class, they had enough income to pay what was not handled by insurance. But not being rich, that meant a heavy financial strain. After Jeff's broken bones healed, the family needed to bring him to a hospital closer to home. That meant us. Someone at their church loaned them an RV to serve as an ambulance, and a nurse volunteered to manage Jeff's IV for the trip. That saved money. Entering through Admissions, the mother told me, would avoid any fees the ER might charge.

People in a coma are never easy, and Jeff was particularly difficult. Almost daily, he'd become upset, with his heart racing at 180 beats per minute and his blood pressure skyrocketing. It's all too easy to see such troublesome patients as less than people, and I struggled with that. To counter that, I talked to him, trying to imagine him listening. Was Jeff aware of his surroundings and merely locked in, unable to communicate? His mother thought so, and that might explain why he became upset.

Long term, there's a danger that such patients will be devalued and moved out of sight. They become discards, cared for only by the lowliest staff, and then only when nothing else needs doing. Worse still, neglected and behind closed curtains or doors, they can become the victims of sexual abuse.

Something else happened with Jeff. As a teaching hospital, we trained nursing students. Most took someone easy as their one-and-only patient despite my efforts to get them to take a patient more demanding. "When your graduate, nursing won't be this easy," I would warn them.

One day, a nursing student was exceptionally bold, and I was delighted when she decided to take Jeff. He would keep her busy, I thought, and take a load off me. More than busy, it turned out. Fed formula through an NG tube, he had an enormous stool, although fortunately not smelly. She's going to be a nurse, I told myself, and needs to learn this. I helped, but made her do the messy part.

Yes, I was being thick-headed again. I was as callous and indifferent to her feelings, as I'd been uneasy about giving Mimi a sponge bath. That illustrates an important point. In hospitals, embarrassment issues are often covered over rather than discussed and resolved. With no thought for the frustrations of that fresh, young nursing student, I forced her to handle a doubly difficult situation—both poop and undress. And why not? I knew no better. No one had taught me how to deal with similar situations, so I had nothing to teach. She and I just blundered along.

The result with Jeff—a procedure clumsy and hastily done—was similar to how the nurse I was working with handled Don's sickle cell treatment, and how I might have coped with Mimi's bath had I not been rescued by a fellow assistant. None of those situations were handled well because issues linked to embarrassment—either of patients or staff—are so rarely discussed.

In the next chapter we'll explore why staff have these difficult-to-express feelings.

21. Scared Ginny

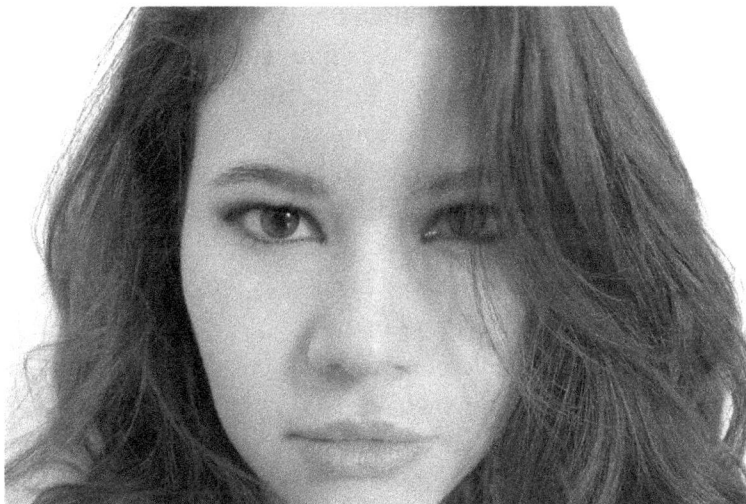

One mid-afternoon on Teens, I was with a girl in the far corner of a room on A cluster, looking away from the other three girls as usual. A specialty nurse who did infection control on central lines came in to care for Ginny, the girl nearest the entrance. She was a dark-haired, sixteen-year-old with bone cancer. To treat her, a central line entered her chest on the upper-right.

Understandably glum, Ginny wasn't talkative, so the nurse started a conversation with me. When I turned around to answer, I saw Ginny with her gown crumpled around her waist. I looked away as fast as I could and asked myself, as if talking to the nurse: "Why did you do that? Ginny lost half of her left arm to cancer. She has that central line for chemotherapy, so her cancer doesn't kill her. She doesn't need me looking at her."

Ginny agreed. Before I looked away, I saw fear in her eyes. Even before the nurse had drawn my attention, she'd been worried about my presence. Still worse, she knew the nurse had opened up a conversation that might have gone on. I could have continued to talk, as that nurse no doubt intended. I might have walked over and began asking about the procedure. If I had, my interest would have been bogus. Hem-Onc handled its own central lines, so I'd helped nurses do the same procedure enough times I could have done it myself. Instead, I turned away, said nothing more, and stalled the care of the patient I was with until the nurse left. I was that angry.

That incident with Ginny raises two questions. The first I stress in *Hospital Gowns*. Why do patients like her allow themselves to be exposed even though they don't like it? She could have insisted that the top of her gown merely be lowered a few inches. That would have been enough for the nurse to do her work. She could have held the gown up herself. That would have worked too. I asked myself that many times, although I knew the answer. Hospitals don't create a climate where avoiding embarrassment is welcomed. Patients are intimidated into inaction. That's bad.

The second question is one I stress here. Why do staff create those situations? Why, for instance, did that nurse get me to turn around? She wasn't being mean. Specialty nurses like her were caring and competent. I appreciated how they patiently answered even the stupidest of my questions.

For the reason, I need look no further than my own behavior. For me it wasn't meanness. It was just not thinking. I was as bad as the female staff I worked with, doing precisely what I complained about. When the patient was a boy, I behaved much like that central-line nurse did with Ginny. Exposing teen guys, I seemed to think, was no big deal. Don in the previous chapter was one illustration, as was Jeff. To illustrate that, in *Hospital Gowns* I describe two patients with much in common, Lenny and Jennie. Notice the distinctions I made between them. That's where the problem lies.

Lenny was about seventeen and had been in the ICU following a motorcycle accident that resulted in a severe head injury. He came to Teens because he'd recovered enough—sitting up, looking around, and being aware his surroundings—that he no longer needed the ICU. Since at first he wasn't quite ready for rehabilitative therapy, we gave him basic care but no more.

After a few days, I felt Lenny had improved enough that he should be transferred to Rehab. But because he still wasn't talking, no one else seemed to notice. I decided on a bold move. Suspecting the nurse wouldn't agree, I waited until she went to lunch to walk him to our bath. From the way he smiled and rolled about in the tub, he obviously loved it. He'd not had a real bath in weeks. He also kept his head above the water, which was the point I wanted to make. He was no vegetable. He simply couldn't talk.

When the nurse returned, she saw Lenny was missing and wanted to know why. With as much innocence as I could fake, I told her he was taking a bath. Her reaction suggested she thought I intended to drown him to free up a bed. I had to show him happily bathing, before she relented. The good news was that, while he was in that tub, his physician came by, saw how well he was doing, and decided to transfer him that afternoon. My scheme was a success. But notice how comfortable I felt about showing Lenny to that nurse. That's indifference to same-sex nudity.

The other incident involved Jennie, another patient in need of therapy. In *Hospital Gowns* I left out a critical detail to make the parallel greater for the teen girls who would be reading it. What I said was true, but what I left out was that Jenny was my patient on the medical unit. She was only six, and thus on the cusp of when children become modest. The lesson I intended still applies.

Jennie had juvenile arthritis. I'd cared for her a few months earlier when she'd been first diagnosed. Then it took an expert to see her difficulties. Now, even I could tell she was developing serious mobility problems. In someone that young, that's terribly sad. Still worse, she was a trim, athletic girl who would have grown up active in sports. Now her entire life would be one long struggle just to be able to walk. Again, you see why I hated auto-immune diseases.

Jennie was scheduled for physical therapy at 8 a.m. Before she went, she wanted a hot bath. Much like I did when I took that nurse to see Lenny bathing, the nurse I was working with saw no problem with my handling the girl's bath. At shift change, everyone was busy, so I couldn't pass the task on. The nurse also wanted me to stay with Jennie, but I persuaded her that the girl could be trusted to use a call light. I could see no reason—short of sheer necessity—why I should hang around while a girl of any age bathed.

I was right. Jenny did use the call light to summon me when she wanted to get out, and all went well over the next several days while she had her therapy. As with Lenny, who was so delighted to bathe that he didn't care who came around, Jennie had no problem with me helping her. The modesty of each isn't the issue here. The issue lies in my attitudes. I had no problem showing a tub-bound Lenny to a female nurse. He was a guy like me and thus no big deal. But I felt uncomfortable with how Jennie might feel with me helping her into a tub. She was a girl and that mattered.

That's the essence of the problem we face here—these dreadfully two-sided and typically under-discussed responses to embarrassing situations. We need to understand why that's true.

First, there's our upbringing as men and women. Recall my memorable seventh-grade experience. I was standing at the corner of the gym waiting for the bell to ring, when a girl in my class who was showering heard me and spoke up. Why do I remember that brief conversation but none of the hundreds of times I showered with others guys in high school and college? Because she was not only a girl, she was one of the prettiest in our class. In the twelfth grade, she'd be voted "Senior Beauty" as well as "Most Intelligent." Talking with her was special, hence my recall. That distinction lies at the heart of this problem.

Second, there's the training that every doctor and nurse receives. It invariably includes desensitization to what most people find distressing: open wounds, body fluids, and nudity. That's necessary. Emergency rooms couldn't function if their doctors and nurses fainted at the sight of blood. As an EMT, I received similar training. With open wounds and body fluids, that works well enough. All it needs to counter is the yuck factor.

With nudity, unfortunately, that training is less successful, in part because it deals with our deep-seated sexuality and in part because the two-sided aspect to desensitization isn't dealt with as openly and effectively as it should. The ease with which staff cope with same-sex nudity enables them to fake situations involving opposite-sex nudity. But faking does not mean coping well. Making matters worse, the stress that formal training places on "if you're professional, this doesn't affect you," creates a powerful incentive to conceal feelings and get by, however poorly.

Recall the nurses I've mentioned, as well as my own frustrations with post-op girls. Having cared for numerous small children, I could do bedpan placement perfectly. I had no problem faking professionalism. But even placing those bedpans without consciously seeing anything didn't change the fact that I couldn't regard a pretty sixteen-year-old girl as if she were a six-year-old boy. My coping was delayed until I could discover a better technique, one I should have been taught as a matter of course.

Third, that lopsided professionalism, as taught in medical and nursing schools, carries over into work. The result in a strange contrast. I've always been amazed at how easily female nurses could discuss embarrassing procedures with me. A labor-and-delivery nurse I dated liked to talk about her work: shaving groins, scrubbing for cesareans, and snipping tubal ligations. One night, a Hem-Onc nurse told me—in graphic detail—how at twelve her doctors had corrected her too-small urethra. I thought, "I can't believe she is telling me this." Nurses are amazing in their candor.

Unfortunately, that openness about procedures doesn't always carry over into embarrassing situations involving patients. While I was frustrated with those post-op bedpans, I consoled myself with an outlandish solution. Maybe, I told myself, I could find a girl who'd let me try different placement techniques until I discovered one that worked. Was that crazy? Yes, but not as crazy as it seems. Remember, those girls had no problem with my doing the procedure several times over several days. This would have just meant those several times came all at once.

Why did I consider that? Because the alternative seemed even crazier from my perspective. That would have been to ask the nurse I was working with if she knew a bedpan technique less intrusive than 'deliver my baby.' Asking her would have suggested that I wasn't "professional." That seemed impossible. Professional pride gets us into a lot of trouble.

Fourth, there are our emotional reactions to embarrassing situations. Our reactions that are often a complex blend of how we feel about a situation combined with how we think our patients feel. I've described those in the chapters about flopping gowns, bedpans, linen changes, and gown changes.

Those feelings confuse us because undress in the opposite sex is both appealing and guilt-inducing. Those feelings, our training implicitly suggests, are most unprofessional. We're supposed regard what happens as of no more significance than drinking coffee. Since that's unlikely, the result is an emotional conflict made all the worse by the fact that those feelings get covered up rather than dealt with openly. Problems that aren't faced, then fester and create additional trouble.

That's why I've been so direct in this book. I want to bring those issues into the sunshine and stress the harm that can result when situations are handled badly, as with Ginny. I want to point out the relaxed feelings and even good humor can exist when embarrassing situations are handled well. People in medicine and nursing should take embarrassment seriously *and* lighten up enough to discuss what is often treated as unmentionable.

Skittishness is one unfortunate result of those confused feelings. You saw that with me on the first day when those helpless post-op girls came under my care. I wanted to make them all wear undies or, failing that, to walk around looking at the floor. And yes, you're right. I didn't *show* my skittishness. I knew that would be unprofessional. Besides, my innate sense of calm and control no matter what carried me through. I'd learned that well on Hem-Onc, where the stresses were enormous. I coped, but not as well as I should.

Another response is the opposite of skittishness—aggression. As I mentioned earlier, embarrassment often results in staff moving quickly so patients have no opportunity to resist. I saw nurses do that with teen guys and understood why. Even sick, those boys were stronger. Moving quickly also reduced the tension a nurse feels Unfortunately, those boys felt differently. That was why they hid under their sheets. They really did feel under siege.

Aggression was never my problem. The girls were so cooperative, I didn't need to bully. I also knew that aggression might make me look bad, perhaps even like a sexual predator. I was also fortunate. I'd spent sixteen months caring for frightened children. I knew how to build trust. Win trust, and you get cooperation. What worked with little kids, also worked with those girls.

All is not lost. Staff don't need to skew wildly from skittishness to aggression. They can steer between the two, making work go better and leaving patients happier. That's best illustrated by those amazing gown changes. As I enjoy reminding you, they were my biggest success. It isn't often that I could get my bored, eager-to-go-home patients to smile, and yet I did.

Notice what happened. As soon as I discovered a girl's gown needed changing, I drew the curtain around her bed. In a room filled with girls, that was saying, "Get ready, in just a minute you're going to be totally naked." No skittishness there. Why did that work? Because being skittish would have delivered the wrong message, telling her, "This is so awful, I feel guilty doing it to you." Nervousness creates fear. Confidence says, "Relax, I done this lots of times. You'll like what happens." By hinting the change might be fun, some even saw it as a girlish adventure much like my seventh-grade friend: "Can he really not embarrass me?"

Was I being too aggressive then? No, when I went for a clean gown, I deliberately took care not to hurry. That gave the girl—who had ample reason to wonder—time to refuse. Being pushy, hurrying her along so quickly that she didn't have time to protest, would convey a different fear, "This is so awful, I must make you do it." Neither was good, and neither proved necessary.

Success with one girl then made me more confident with the next. A girl, looking around at those drawn curtains and down at a gown knowing she has not a scrap of clothing beneath, nevertheless thought, "Well, he *seems* to think this will go well. Maybe I should trust him." Success brought that beautiful smile, as events confirmed her hope. The result was fun for both of us.

Yes, I was fortunate. A yucky gown provided ample motivation to cooperate. Also, we hadn't just met. I'd been caring for her for hours if not days, and she had seen me interacting with other girls. Most important of all, my confidence was rooted in reality. I *knew* I could fulfill my implied promise that all would go well.

With gown changes, I was fortunate in another way. Look-in-the-eyes meant no touching or seeing. Not all procedures are that easy. A female nurse placing a urine catheter in a man must touch. A male physician doing a pelvic exam on a woman must look. Those are unavoidable. In many cases, they're also dealing with a patient they've only just met. How can staff make a procedure go better?

I can't speak as an expert, but I can adapt what I have learned. The details may differ, but not the basic principles. Apply them, and all will go better. What seems awkward at first, will get better when you acquire the knack.

First, show you care. With those Hem-Onc kids, the core problem was all the misery created by our chemotherapy. Did I have to stand alongside them holding a bucket when they vomited? No, most of the time I didn't. Those kids could have managed it either themselves or with help from their parents. But by doing that, I showed I liked them. They picked up on that.

I did much the same with those post-op girls. By lunch on the first day with that first group, I was applying those three guidelines. I was careful to follow them thereafter, no matter how tired. Did I have to do that? Probably not. As miserably hot as their room was, most girls would have continued to roll on their sides unless my behavior had been downright creepy. But merely being tolerable wasn't good enough. I wanted them comfortable. They picked up on that and trusted me. Learn ways to make patients comfortable.

Second, apply the ten percent principle. Ninety percent of the benefits often come from the last ten percent of effort. That's particularly true in hospitals, where patients see that added effort.

Toward the end of summer, I considered slacking off. All was going so well, I told myself, doing less would change little. Given our heavy workload, the effort I put into those post-op girls was exhausting. Even if I became sloppy, I realized, they weren't going to cower beneath their sheets like our boys. But after some thought, I decided to keep up the added effort. Why? Because I liked the results. I enjoyed hints that some girls actually liked have a guy going out of his way to reduce their embarrassment, rather than a woman who might be too relaxed.

Third, set high standards. Despite the pressures, I maintained high standards. I quit doing linen changes because they were hated and I knew no way to make them better. I did gown changes because girls loved them. I wasn't trying to just get by. I wanted to make my patients as comfortable as possible.

Fourth, be adaptable. All patients aren't alike, so leave room for differences. Yes, Min's modesty frustrated me. Flipping her over was difficult enough. Doing so while adjusting her covering sheet was even more so. Yet I did my best. At the opposite extreme, the casualness of those first post-op girls frustrated me. Yet I did what they wanted. In both cases, I let patients be themselves. I adapted to them as much as possible.

Fifth, relax and trust patients. Never forget that almost all patients want their hospital stay to go as well as possible. That means they're willing to adjust as long as what they're expected to accept seems reasonable. Work to make that so and don't forget that trying will make up for not being perfect.

Sixth, be confident even under pressure. Once you develop the necessary skills, don't let the awkward situations that arise rattle you or make you feel guilty, and that's true even with catheters or pelvic exams. Do your best and be content with that. Your patients will see your confidence and relax.

To illustrate, I'll close with an incident that in *Hospital Gowns* that I call "Miss Buns and the Wet Hens." It came near the end of my time on Teens and shows in an amusing way how unflappable I'd become by then. It was also the only time a room full of girls turned on me.

After morning report, my first decision was whether to check the vital signs for the boys or girls. I usually determined that by which room had the most talking. That gave those in the other room a few more minutes sleep. On this particular day, I checked the boys first.

When I walked into the girls room there was Miss Buns, about fifteen or so, lying on her tummy with her sheet kicked down and the back of her gown open to the warm morning sun. How typical of our nurses, I thought. When the night nurse made her last check before we arrived, she no doubt found that cute. They were like that.

Not cute for me though. I was in a bind. The other three girls were glaring at me like angry wet hens. Good for you, I thought, but why didn't you cover her up before I came? I could tell they wanted me to scurry away, but I knew that if I didn't get their vital signs done before breakfast, my morning would be a mess. "No girls," I sent them a silent message, "I'm not looking at Miss Buns, but I'm also not leaving. I'll get your vital signs and leave hers for later."

There was another issue. Miss Buns was visible from the door and in just a few minutes the boys would be up. I knew that the instant I left, a hen would hurry to her bed, and that proved true.

When I delivered breakfast trays a few minutes later, Miss Buns was sitting up and doing her best to appear prim and proper. Shortly afterward she left for a clinic appointment. Before long, the three wet hens calmed down, assured I wasn't a Peeping Mike after all. That didn't surprise me.

How should we feel about Miss Buns? Yes, she was a silly girl to sleep like that when a room filled with boys her age was only six steps away. She was also the only patient I cared for who displayed genuine, outside-a-hospital embarrassment, blushing when I came into her room for the second time. She was blaming herself, as indeed she ought.

Hospitals rarely create embarrassing situations where patients have reason to blame themselves. Most situations are driven by necessity, such as bedpans. For a few, the necessity seem dubious enough that patients legitimately get ticked off. That's those linen changes. In neither does the patient think, "This is all my fault." They're right. If it's badly done, it is the hospital's fault. Staff need to be better trained and more careful.

Most intriguing for me were situations where a patient was delighted by what at first glance seemed embarrassing. My gown changes were one example. They were done so perfectly, the girls smiled, thinking: "I *really* can trust this guy." Many also smiled when I pinned up the back of their gowns. That too made sense. I wasn't embarrassing them. My status as staff did give me a little freedom. Instead, I was keeping them from discovering to their horror why our teen boys were giggling at them.

So do your work so well that patients enjoy what they might have otherwise disliked. Use distracting talk, a towel, sheer speed, a cautious approach, looking them in the eyes, or whatever to say, "Relax, I know what I'm doing. I'm looking out for you."

Ah, but there's another situation, one that comes when a patient blames someone on staff for unnecessary embarrassment. That's next. You might also try guessing who the cause of the embarrassment is.

22. FURIOUS KAY

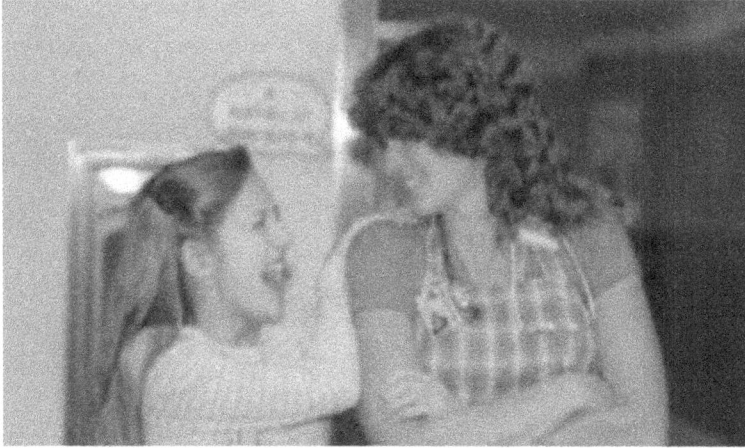

I mentioned our nurses looked like cheerleaders. That's one on the right, so you can see for yourself. Next to her is one of the two girls that I called "the twins." She is Kay, full of zest and a special favorite of mine. Her feelings about me were a bit more complex, as we'll soon see.

I called them twins, not because they were related, but because both were in their early twenties and came in at the same time. The picture hints at why. Notice how short Kay is. The nurse is about five-feet-four, so she's under five feet. In a picture I took just seconds earlier, she's waving exuberantly at me. That picture shows what her stylish clothing usually hid, an enlarged upper rib cage.

You may have guessed that she has cystic fibrosis. She's short because of nutritional issues. Her rib cage is large due to exhausting days spent battling lung infections. To keep her well, about every two months she came in for a 'tune up' with her twin.

Some medical history will help. Today, many of those with cystic fibrosis live well into their thirties. But in the past, only a few lived past childhood. Like my cousin Beth, they died young. That was changing when I knew Kay. When the twins appeared, I was troubled by questions I dare not ask: "How many were in their tune-up program when it began?" Now there were but two. "How did that feel?" Not good, I suspected. They were the survivors.

Why did I consider Kay special? Like many who worked in hospitals, I appreciated fighters, meaning patients who refused to let their illness dictate their lives. They made my work feel more worthwhile. One of Kay's doctors told me patients who fought the hardest usually lived the longest.

As you can see from the picture, Kay had that fighting spirit in abundance. Notice that she's attractively dressed. No washed-out hospital clothing for her. She brought hers from home. She's wearing makeup too and has beautifully done hair. Most of our teens would lie in bed until nine or ten, and the girls did not bother with makeup or hair. Kay would be up, tastefully dressed and pretty, when I arrived at seven. That impressed me.

Ah, but as much as I liked Kay, from our first day on she treated me with disdain. As you see, she was friendly with nurses, so I decided the trouble was that I was a guy. That confused me. Embarrassment wasn't an issue. All I did was take her vital signs and bring her a meal tray. In *Hospital Gowns* I suggested that the embarrassment she experienced during physical therapy was transferred to me. At any rate, I admired her grit and determination too much to be upset. For all her seeming chilliness, I liked her.

Then something happened to alter our relationship. During one of Kay's visits, she shared a room with Ida, a sixteen-year-old girl with severe juvenile arthritis, who was in for physical therapy. One afternoon, Ida needed to void, so I helped her walk, ever-so-slowly, to our toilet. When she finished, I walked her back.

At this point, it helps to understand that I never rushed patients. If walking was painful, I didn't hurry them. If they wanted to talk, I listened, no matter how busy. To make up for lost time, when I wasn't with a patient, I moved lightning fast.

That day, I had orders to monitor Ida's urine output, so as soon as she was back in bed, I darted for the urine collection bin I'd placed in her toilet bowl. As I opened the door, there was a scream of outrage. Kay must have needed to go really badly. While I'd been walking Ida back to bed, she had slipped in. I let the door fall shut, mumbled an apology, and hurried away.

Kay was furious. The next day, Ms. Ding Dong called me in. Keep in mind what typically happened at our meetings. Convinced our nursing staff were lazy or incompetent, she could be nasty. I kept a low profile, but on one occasion, I felt her wrath in a way that'll help you understand the strangeness of this meeting about Kay.

Ms. Ding Dong had gone through our nursing notes, digging up what she thought was dirt on us. Mine was so absurd, I felt flattered by what she'd come up with. If that's all she can find, I told myself, I must be doing very well indeed.

Tad was a husky, seventeen-year-old guy and, although quiet, he wasn't withdrawn like most teen boys. His battle with bone cancer had reconciled him to us. On this visit, he was getting cisplatin, a chemotherapy "drug from hell." Unless carefully managed, it causes severe renal damage. I knew it well from Hem-Onc, and nothing would keep me from following the treatment protocol to the letter. That meant a fast IV and forcing a void every two hours. If his treatment had been up to me, I'd have doubled that IV rate, carefully monitored him for fluid overload, and made him void every hour. Did I mention I hated that drug? Cisplatin makes ordinary chemotherapy seem like sweetness and light.

Needless to say, I handled Tad's treatment to perfection, enjoying a rare opportunity to use skills I'd acquired on Hem-Onc. Since all went well, I recorded his on-time voids much like his nurse was recording his high IV rate. Ah, but Ms. Ding Dong, in her zeal to dig up dirt, attacked me for not elaborating in those notes. That was nonsense, I thought. Nothing wrong meant nothing to log—that was standard procedure. If anything had gone bad, rest assured I would have raised bloody hell. On Hem-Onc, to get the four a.m. void, I often had to wake up the resident and get an order for Lasix.

Do you get the point? Ms. Ding Dong enjoyed finding fault even when her charges were bogus. That's why the way she handled Kay's complaint angered me. Contrary to our other meetings, she wasn't out to get me. She had not even done a through investigation. As soon as I offered my explanation, the issue was over. She was eager to put it aside. That's all too typical of how hospitals handle sex-tinged issues.

"Hey, wait," I felt like saying. "Aren't you going to check my story? Will you see if Ida really did have an order to monitor her fluids? Will you make sure I recorded that void? After all, Kay is pretty. I might have seen her go into the toilet and deliberately burst in on her."

Yes, I know the last is nonsense, given all the toilet visits and bedpans I had to handle, but I think you get the point. My guilt wasn't even being considered. Ms. Ding Dong *wanted* me innocent. Normally crabby, she *wanted* to let me off, and I knew why. For issues like that, hospitals are often disturbingly eager to take a staff member's word over that of a patient. Fearful of the legal consequences, they're not fair or objective. Patients suffer, and creeps on staff have little to fear as long as they keep the situation 'he said, she said.' Even if caught in the act, there's often a cover-up. If there's a lawsuit, a cover-up is even more likely.

The medical literature reflects that bias. While writing *Hospital Gowns,* a research librarian and I found only one article in numerous medical and nursing databases that touched on embarrassment. That was one about "integrity issues" for Iranian women in Iranian hospitals. We did find a related one, although not about embarrassment. It looked at situations where a patient made an accusation of a sexual nature against staff. What those writing the article regarded as good news, I saw as dreadful. Typically, in disputes with little or no evidence other than conflicting testimonies, the courts favored the hospital. That's why hospitals see little reason to reform. They may be forced to change, however, particularly after scandals where what happened was captured on smartphones. "It was recorded" will settle a 'he said, she said' dispute.

That's why, when I tell teen girls how to deal with creepy behavior in *Hospital Gowns,* I'm clear that they should not expect support from an administration getting legal advice that say, "Admit nothing. We may end up in court." I tell those girls how to work around an often dysfunctional system. Here's a short summary.

First, take your suspicions seriously. A good guy, I tell them, will go out of his way to make you feel comfortable. If you're not, he's probably a creep testing you for weakness. Don't worry about his feelings. He doesn't deserve your kindness. Coldly drive him away by any means. That may be all the protection you need. You've demonstrated you're not weak and won't be an easy victim.

Second, assume the worse and prepare. Take notes of suspicious events to use later as evidence. Nothing scares lawyers like written documentation (or text messages with a time stamp). Once you have evidence, talk to your parents. If trouble develops, you'll need their support. If you're in a room with other girls, ask them to watch. Their testimony may prove valuable. If you've got a smartphone or other recording device, look for opportunities to use it. Recording video or audio can tilt the case heavily in your favor. If this goes legal, you'll need hard evidence. It will also make a hospital's lawyers more willing to settle out of court, sparing you considerable hassle and uncertainty.

Third, take your suspicions to a kind nurse, but don't try to accomplish too much. Stress your comfort, rather than making the issue so serious she has to take it up with administration. Yes, in the long-term something needs to be done about that creep, but for now focus on protecting yourself. Part of a nurse's job is to fit care to the patient. She can make adjustments to keep that guy out of your room. If your situation comes before administrators, they may go into a defensive mode that's unlikely to do you any immediate good.

Fourth, if there's a guy on staff you trust, explain your concerns to him. He's more likely to take you seriously than anyone else. Who knows, he may even confront that guy directly, man-to-creep, and he won't bother to be nice. I know, I came close to just such a confrontation myself.

During my entire ten months working days on Teens, I was its only male staff, although for a time there was a married guy working evenings. On a single occasion during that busy summer the nursing administration floated a male to us. Within minutes, I knew this Mr. Lurk was a creep. He seemed suspiciously eager to linger in the room with those adorable but ill-clad post-op girls. I'd worked hard to ensure they felt comfortable. I was not going to let him ruin that. Alas, Mr. Lurk was spared a clash with me. Only a few minutes after arriving, he was sent elsewhere. I never saw him again, so hopefully I wasn't the only one to notice his behavior.

What would I have done if Mr. Lurk had remained assigned to Teens? I'd have done nothing as slow and uncertain as an incident report. I'd have taken him aside and told him, "I know what you intend, and I won't permit it. Those girls are my patients. You will not enter their room—not now or ever."

Doing that, I would be displaying professionalism and a healthy masculinity. Professionally, those girls were my patients. I decided who provided their basic care. Unfortunately, I doubt Mr. Lurk understood professionalism. That was why he needed a sterner message, the same that I and other guys sent creeps while traveling. "Stay away or suffer the consequences."

Some will say, "You can't do that. What will result?" Most likely, the creepy behavior will end quickly and without further ado. The girls I traveled with were never hassled, while Miss Europe and I enjoyed that Jerusalem concert. In hospitals, small problems become costly because informal, effective solutions are rejected and only clumsy bureaucratic ones are permitted. That makes no sense. Hospitals should *encourage* staff to act informally before a potential problem becomes a disaster. They'll save themselves a sea of troubles. Better to prevent than to be sued.

Intimidation works, because creeps are cowards who see women as prey. Stand up to them, and they scurry away. Nor is that necessarily masculine. The next chapter describes how I saw nurses use similarly bold techniques. Acting informally has other advantages. First, calling someone a pervert openly or by implication isn't slander if no one else is present. Second, keeping a confrontation private forces on the creep the onus of making it an administrative issue. That he's unlikely to do, since it would call attention to him.

What about the opposite scenario, one where I might stand accused? Several times a day I was in situations that might have become messy. I might do something behind drawn curtains and deny it. I might do nothing, but be unfairly charged. Only she and I would know. I never felt that was a problem, because I trusted these girls and they felt the same. Even Kay's anger was about what I'd done not what I'd intended to do. But my situation was not universal. Hospitals need policies that let staff to protect themselves when they suspect they're being setup for an accusation. They should be able to ask another staff for assistance and witnessing.

Now back to Kay. I liked her too much to get mad. Hospital-savvy, she knew when she removed Ida's bin, I'd be back. While the doors of the toilet weren't lockable, she knew how to grab the door handle. For all her initial fury, I knew she wasn't going to stay angry. She had her dignity—oodles of it—and our little accident had insulted it. That was all.

Indeed, as I look back, I realize that from then on, Kay began to warm to me. You see that in the picture at the start of this chapter. She was showing off for my camera and delighted by my attention. I think I now understand her aloofness. Yes, it was because I was a guy. Notice all the efforts she made to be attractive—getting up early to shower, put on makeup, and dress well. She made herself pretty because, perhaps even more than most other girls her age, she wanted guys to find her attractive. She wanted their attention.

But there was this dreadful curse—cystic fibrosis. How many times had she met a guy who seemed interested until he discovered that? She may have been forced to tell one, "You don't want to like me. I don't have long to live. You'll only get hurt."

Her desire to be liked wasn't just about boys. Look at that picture again. Notice the body language. I took that picture at just the right moment. Her posture is saying to the nurse, "Please come close to me for this picture Mike wants to take." But notice too the dramatic contrast. Her nurse is turning away with her arms crossed. That's saying, "No, I don't want to get close. You're going to die, and I don't want to get hurt." Yet at the same time, the nurse is yielding to Kay's efforts. That is why she's turning her head toward Kay and smiling. She's saying, "Well, maybe just this once." That's easy to understand. Our nurses were kind.

Kay's feelings for me resemble those for her nurse but were complicated by the fact that I was a guy. She feared to get close to me because—even though she had no romantic interest—I represented yet another guy who, if she made an effort, might reject her. That explains why she warmed after our toilet incident. I didn't get angry, so maybe I could be trusted not to run away. She didn't know that I'd spent sixteen months liking little kids, some of who were doomed to die. I could do the same with her.

Alas, the story doesn't end there. Some of our patients went to the ICU. If they improved, they typically came to us before being discharged, but a few died two floors up. On their own initiative, the ICU nurses were great. They came down and told us when someone we knew died. Otherwise, we might have never heard.

One day, an ICU nurse told me the bad news. Kay had been admitted directly to the ICU with a terrible lung infection, one that proved resistant to antibiotics. After several days of feverish struggle, she died. Her long and valiant battle was over.

Looking back, I have regrets. I wish I'd responded better to her belated effort at friendship. If we'd talked, I could have told her about my cousin, as well as how impressed as I was by her grit and determination. Sadly, that was not to be. Opportunities not seized are often lost forever. At best, I can remind myself that she discovered I wanted to be her friend. That was something. I can also ensure that she's not forgotten by writing about her.

Thus far, I've dealt with embarrassing situations that were sometimes handled well and sometimes clumsily. For both, there was no malice. Nurses did not intend to be mean when they left those barely dressed post-op girls with me. Caring for them was simply my job. Nor was I being mean when I did something similar with the boys. That's just how embarrassing issues were handled. There weren't many practical alternatives to what we were doing, nor was anyone seriously harmed in the great majority of cases. Our patients understood that a hospital isn't a five-star hotel.

But other possibilities exist. Imagine a situation where there are those who don't mean well, particularly when the patient in question is an exceptionally pretty girl. Matters can go badly. That's next.

23. LOST CARINA

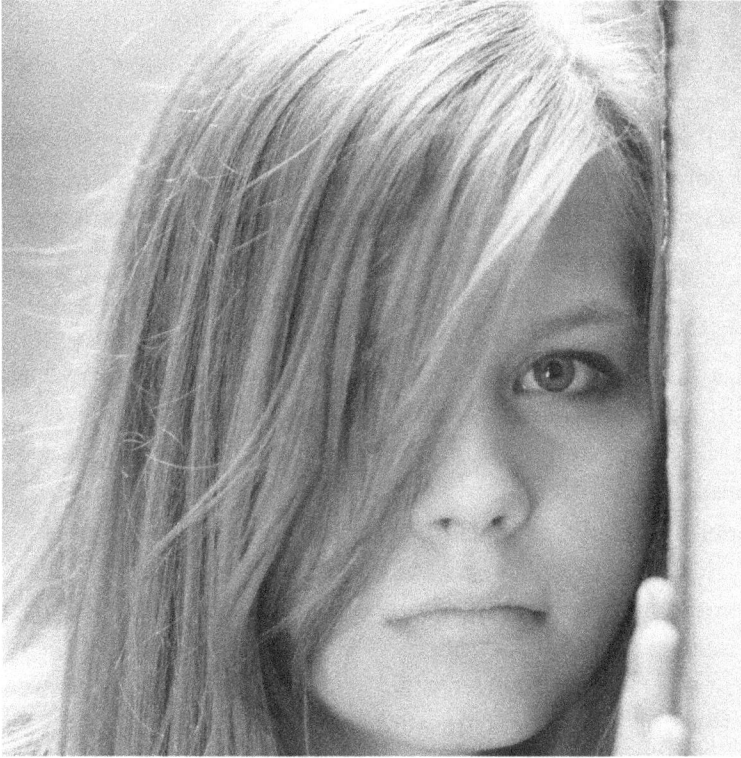

First, a brief disclaimer. At times, I joked to myself that, if I'd gotten out of line caring for these girls, the nurse I was working with would have given me trouble. That was certainly true, although in my case, the nurses probably regarded me as a bit more skittish than I needed to be. I wanted my patients comfortable.

Also, throughout this book, I've done my best to look on the sunny side. I've raised issues, but shown that, with good intentions and abundant thought, they can be managed, particularly when patients and staff work together.

But suppose there were some who roamed a hospital, having less accountability imposed on them than I did. That creates an opportunity for mischief doesn't it? That's the topic of this chapter. Get ready for serious change. We're leaving the sunshine and plunging into darkness. I'd originally written an entire chapter with weak apologies for this misbehavior, but it grew so muddled, I gave up. I'll offer three limp excuses instead.

First, these people weren't the primary malefactors. The greatest blame lay with those in more responsible positions. After all, this was a children's hospital not a crowded metropolitan ER. Dubious staff behavior and worse should have been prevented by firm, written policies. It's difficult imagine a procedure more in need of limits than pelvic exams given to girls as young as twelve. There's simply no excuse this failure, and the blame lay with those in power—the hospital's senior physicians and administrators.

Keep in mind too that, while training about sexually transmitted diseases (STDs) was necessary, it could have been accomplished with a trip to a STD clinic that routinely handled such diseases. Doing the exam on a cynical, forty-year-old prostitute does not raise the same 'do no harm' issues as doing it on a confused girl in her mid-teens. Teaching can't excuse the inexcusable.

Second, their education stressed knowledge over all else. Encyclopedic knowledge is imparted as if that's all that matters. But knowing *only* what is in textbooks blinds to what's not in them and may be more important. In the situation we'll discuss next, the patient's personality mattered far more that the antibiotics treating her. That was where her care went tragically wrong.

Third, they had limited relationships with patients. My work put me in close contact with them. On Hem-On, I cared for seven children all night, and most stayed for weeks. That remained partly true on Teens, particularly with major orthopedic surgeries. In a typical day I might spend half an hour with someone who'd be my patient for a week. That built a relationship.

That was not true for those we discuss here Their work was a whirl of activity. They roved the hospital, rarely spending more than a few minutes with any one patient. And no, I'm not saying that a lack of emotional bonds excuses what they did. But it does offer insight into why this particular young girl could be treated so badly.

Now we turn to that unfortunate day. The patient was Carina, a breathtakingly pretty fifteen-year-old with beautiful light-brown hair. To give you an idea what she looked like, I searched through hundreds of stock photos. The one at the start of this chapter is the closest match in appearance and personality.

I'm not sure how the word spread, but from all over our hospital male residents came to Teens to learn how to do a pelvic exam on the beautiful Carina. Since only one exam was need for a pelvic inflammatory disease (PID) diagnosis, after no less that eight of those intimate, probing exams, the nurse I was working with drove those lecherous doctors-in-training out of the exam room. She was still ticked off when I came back from lunch and was told about what had happened.

This is how the Center for Disease Control defines Carina's PID. It's a dastardly, complication-ridden infection that no sane woman wants to get.

> Pelvic inflammatory disease (PID) refers to infection of the uterus (womb), fallopian tubes (tubes that carry eggs from the ovaries to the uterus) and other reproductive organs that causes symptoms such as lower abdominal pain. It is a serious complication of some sexually transmitted diseases (STDs), especially chlamydia and gonorrhea. PID can damage the fallopian tubes and tissues in and near the uterus and ovaries. PID can lead to serious consequences including infertility, ectopic pregnancy (a pregnancy in the fallopian tube or elsewhere outside of the womb), abscess formation, and chronic pelvic pain.

Take particular note of the possible consequences for Carina. They include never being able to have a child, a life-threatening outside-the-womb pregnancy, and pain that never goes away. This isn't a case of the sniffles. It's a highly destructive infection that can completely wreck a woman's entire life while she's still a teen.

Keep in mind that a PID is not like a cold. It's never really cured. If you've have this infection even once, the internal scaring and other damage will be with you for the rest of your life. Subsequent infections are not only more likely, they increase those risks of sterility, death, and chronic pain. PID is one of the worst infections a woman can get, and that's what this young girl had. She needed to be treated with particular gentleness.

The CDC goes on to stress the special dangers for young girls such as Carina, warning that: "Sexually active women in their childbearing years are most at risk, and those under age 25 are more likely to develop PID than those older than 25. This is partly because the cervix of teenage girls and young women is not fully matured, increasing their susceptibility to the STDs that are linked to PID." Ponder this—if those risks exist as late as twenty-five, imagine how terrible they are at fifteen. That was Carina's situation. Yet as a patient at our children's hospital, she was being treated as the pelvic exam equivalent of a CPR mannequin.

Sadly, it was all too easy to see how Carina had been lured into the destructive behavior that led to her infection. I cared for her during her entire stay. I've never met anyone else who had less of a self in the sense of having a will that could say "no." She was soft and passive, which no doubt that added to her attractiveness to men of all sorts, good and evil. But since that was not balanced by any good sense, her softness was making her life a living hell.

In medicine there's a term called 'compliance' that refers to following orders. Carina's problem was that she was all compliance and no resistance. That's why she'd gotten her PID. That was why she let those eager young male residents examine her—legs in stirrups and spread wide—without protest. Her problems clearly went beyond her infection, as terrible as that was. Her personality posed a greater threat to her future happiness than any disease.

Now look at that picture again. I chose it carefully. Carina had that same hopeless look in her eyes. She seemed sad, lost, and lonely—all at once. At fifteen, she seemed to have given up on life.

Carina's issues were different from any other teen girl I cared for. With her, it wasn't what she regarded as embarrassing or as wronging her—which seemed to be almost nothing—but how we, as physicians and staff, should be treating her based on her own best interests. That obviously included making certain she never got another PID. We need to do for her what she couldn't do for herself. We needed to display the good sense she lacked in the hope that, as she grew older, she would mature and grow wiser.

Fortunately, I found myself liking her. The same fragility and vulnerability that attracted sexual predators made me want to protect her.

And she certainly needed protection. She was all compliance and no resistance. She had no self to say, "Do this" or "Don't do that." None at all.

And no, she wasn't quite like Ado Annie Carnes in that delightful Rogers and Hammerstein musical "Oklahoma." If you watch the movie version, Ado is the one who sings:

I heared a lot of stories and I reckon they are true
About how girls're put upon by men.
I know I mustn't fall into the pit,
But when I'm with a feller,
I fergit!
I'm just a girl who cain't say no.

First, because Carina was much prettier, which put her at far greater risk. Ado only had two suitors, and one wanted to marry her. I doubt Carina's false suitors had anything on their minds but sex.

While writing this, I pondered what her life as a ninth-grader must have been like. Did she have a reputation for looseness that meant girls her age resented and shunned her? That would explain her loneliness. Was she passed between bad guys as an easily conquered but quickly discarded sex toy? That seemed likely too. Still worse, none of those guys, having had his way, would admit to his peers that he liked her. That left her feeling lost. Finally, guys who would have treated her kindly were put off by her reputation. That explained her sadness.

Second, unlike Ado in the movie, Carina didn't strike me as lacking intelligence. Despite her absence of willpower, there was something about her that impressed. She had class, and by that I mean that both she and her mother gave every indication of coming from a affluent, well-educated background. If she'd shown up on Teens claiming to be a third-year premed student, we would have believed her. She also looked older than her fifteen years. That made her plight still worse.

Third, I never got the impression she was being swept off her feet by the disease-riddled guys wrecking her life. It was simply a matter of what they wanted, they got. She had no will of her own to be either overwhelmed or broken. She wasn't like Pala, briefly overwhelmed by circumstances, or Tina, desperate to avoid dying. This was far worse. This was her entire life. This was who she was, not what was happening to her.

If you're looking to understand her, consider what some call "daddy hunger." Her father never visited while she was with us and seemed absent from her life. That left her vulnerable to attention from any male, however destructive.

The slit in the back of Carina's gown illustrates her vulnerability. Most girls had the good sense to take care of that themselves before they left their room. The few who forgot were happy when I penned it up. I'd spared them embarrassment. Carina was like neither. Day after day, she'd leave her room, the bright red panties she'd brought from home flashing with each step. Yet when I would catch her and pin that slit up, her response was—well nothing.

That left me dumbfounded. No other girl I recall wore red. No other girl was indifferent to exposing her undies to our teen boys. In one sense, Carina was being sexually provocative, very much so. Yet in another sense, she wasn't. Women who intend to look sexy, project it in how they walk. Carina was certainly attractive, yet she radiated no sexiness. For her, sex was little more than what men wanted.

Later, I asked myself how she would have responded if, following our three-day rule, I'd walked her to our shower and undressed her. Any other girl in her situation would have screamed in protest, pointedly telling me she could handle that herself. I doubt Carina would have done anything. Fortunately, that idea only came to me after she was discharged. Also, I'm joking to make a point.

Carina's core problem was her inability to say no, and not just as a laugh line in a musical. That said, the answer to Carina's weakness was not that different from the one for Ado in the movie "Oklahoma." That's where her story turns from sad to tragic. Ado was growing up in a small town in Oklahoma during the late nineteenth century and was being treated with a common sense that's as old as the hills. Carina had the misfortune to be in what is today one of the top ten children's hospitals in country and receiving what passes for good medicine today.

To understand what the hospital might have done for Carina, I'll tell you about a situation a friend of mine is in. For years he has befriended a young black man we'll call Carl, whose life is a mess.

Carl lost his job with the public school system and is overweight. He keeps talking about going back to school and getting a marketable skill, but never acts on that vague wish, even when he's out of work with nothing else to do. He gets ripped off every time he buys a used car. As my friend pointed out, the guy never had a father to teach him about cars and his mother, living on welfare, never owned one. He was, just as I said, a mess.

But those were the least of his worries. His real problem came when Jill, a fourteen-year-old girl he'd known from his former school job, got in touch with him. They exchanged sexually tinged messages via cell phone, and he dropped by her house planning to do you-know-what. Keep in mind that he's twenty-seven, only one year shy of twice her age. Did I say he is a mess?

Less than a minute after he arrived at Jill's home, the phone rang. It was the girl's mom informing Carl that, if he wasn't out of her home that instant, she was calling the cops. His troubles didn't end there, with statutory rape not yet having happened. Because his contact was through his former job, the mother got the school district involved, which led to legal action. In his state exchanging digital messages like his with a minor is a felony sex offense. If he'd communicated the same words with notes on paper, it would have been a much less serious misdemeanor. Law has its quirks.

When my friend told me about that, I suspected Carl's life was over. He now had a record as a sex offender that'll stay with him for who knows how long. Since work anywhere near children requires a background check, about the only work he was qualified to do was casual labor in a warehouse or at a construction site, something his weight made impossible. Even worse, that girl's mother has made a mission out of wrecking his life. When his sex-offender status came up for review years later, she prevented it from being revoked. She is a mother with a mission. Of course, she also did him an inadvertent favor. But for her, he might have been charged with statutory rape.

Yes, it is possible to make excuses. My friend did just that. "Hey, this guy goes to a church where the pastor has had six kids by five different women," he said. "It's not like he's had any good male role models in his life." "Yeah, yeah," I answered, "but it's still hard to see why he couldn't see that he was way out of line with a mixed-up girl half his age."

Notice that nothing happened because that clueless fourteen-year-old girl had a very together mother who was making up for what her young daughter lacked. Since the mother was miles away at work when she called, she must have persuaded a neighbor to watch her house and call if any suspicious visitors arrived. The mother was playing a role much like that of a father with a shotgun in "Oklahoma." She was an enforcer saying the "no" that her daughter couldn't say at that age. She was giving her daughter enough time to grow up and acquire good sense before she wrecked her life.

Most important of all, she was doing what good families have always done—protect their most vulnerable members. Thanks to her, perhaps the fourteen-year-old Jill wouldn't get a PID, ending up sterile with constant abdominal pain. Such a mother might be portrayed nastily as a prude in our contemporary, sex-saturated media, but she was a good mom and should to be seen as a heroine.

Nor is there anything new about what Jill's mom was doing. In the eighth chapter of the biblical *Song of Solomon* (1000 B.C.), a young girl's older brothers who play that role. In the poem, the first verse uses poetic imagery to describe a younger sister who is approaching puberty, and the day when she will be "spoken for" in marriage. In the second, a contrast is made between a sister who has a strong will, represented by a wall, whose youthful good looks can be safely enhanced with an appealing "battlement" of silver jewelry (her marriage dowry), with one who is weak and open like a door and needs protecting with sturdy "boards of cedar."

> We have a little sister and she has no breasts. What shall we do for our sister on the day when she is spoken for?
> If she is a wall, we will build on her a battlement of silver, but if she is a door, we will enclose her with boards of cedar.

That's where our modern story turns terribly tragic. Carina had the misfortune to be in a modern hospital following up-to-date treatment protocols. Except for antibiotics to deal with that infection—antibiotics that become less effective with each passing year—she would have been better off being born at almost any other time in history. That's what lies at the heart of her tragedy.

Now back to my situation. I wasn't aware of those verses at the time, but I understood their intent. I took on the role of Carina's big brother. I treated her kindly, but didn't try to get close. She might misinterpret that. I kept a close watch for any contact she might have with males of dubious intent. In ancient terms, I tended those "boards of cedar."

Fortunately, I'd learned something earlier. Working nights, at report an evening nurse told us what she'd just done. One father had been hanging around his daughter's multi-bed room, she suspected, to get a glimpse of little girls when they were undressed. She knew that if she confronted Mr. Creepy Dad, there'd be a clash, security would be called, and a nasty lawsuit might follow. Bad people are often thin-skinned.

She told us what she did instead. Our multi-bed rooms didn't have room for parents, although there was no specific rule forbidding their presence except for no overnight stays. To get rid of Mr. Creepy Dad, she contrived a rule, telling him he couldn't stay more than a few minutes. That forced him to leave. That was brilliant. Hospitals, I will admit, often have too many rules. But their existence can be helpful.

I did much the same for Carina. I took care to keep the slit on her gown pinned, lest that draw the attention of a teen guy who, in a few seconds might pick up on how 'easy' she was. Before he could chat her up and get her phone number, I intended to step in and contrive a non-fraternization policy. Since our boys and girls rarely chatted anyway, that would seem plausible.

My greatest worry, however, was that Dr. Creepy Resident, who'd been part of that original lecherous eight, would return for what he might call "follow-up care." The odds were that no one had assigned him to her, that his own fevered mind had contrived the scheme for dubious reasons.

I was ready for that. Keep in mind my background. On Hem-Onc nights one of my greatest fears was that I'd sense one of our kids was in trouble, but find myself unable to get the treatment altered by an inexperienced night resident. That so bothered me, I'd pondered long and hard how to play hospital power games. I saw that the games rewarded those who remained calm but offered solid reasons for a particular course of action.

So while Dr. Creepy Resident might outrank a mere assistant like me, I had advantages and intended to use them. Carina was my patient, and he was on my turf. To get Carina into that exam room again, he'd have to get past me. That was not going to happen. Since she knew me well, she would do what I said. I could call on our nurses too. They knew what our male residents had done when she was admitted. They'd back me up. All I need do was make a stand.

Blocked that way, Dr. Creepy Resident would almost certainly sulk away. He did not want to draw attention to himself. But if he tried to push, I knew how to push back. Citing how badly Carina been treated on admission, I'd insist that her discharge exam be done by a woman. That was an irrefutably good reason. Applying it would be easy and appropriate. Indeed, some medical arguments are so good, they need only be raised to win. All that is needed is the courage to raise them.

In a similar situation, command the high ground with a good argument, calmly dig in, and force your opponents to attack uphill. Plan your argument carefully and anticipate criticism. Stay cool and let them lose their temper. Win by out-thinking.

Fortunately, neither measure proved necessary. Carina completed her antibiotics and went home. I wasn't happy with the outcome though. As far as I could tell, the only assistance we gave her were those antibiotics. She got no help with her real problems. That illustrates all too well our modern taboos about anything connected with sex, particularly that of teens.

Now for another warning. As dark as this chapter has been, the next will be even worse. The experience it recounts won't involve my patients. It'll be that of a medical student who does not hesitate to refer to what she saw as a "child rape."

24. Horrified Med Student

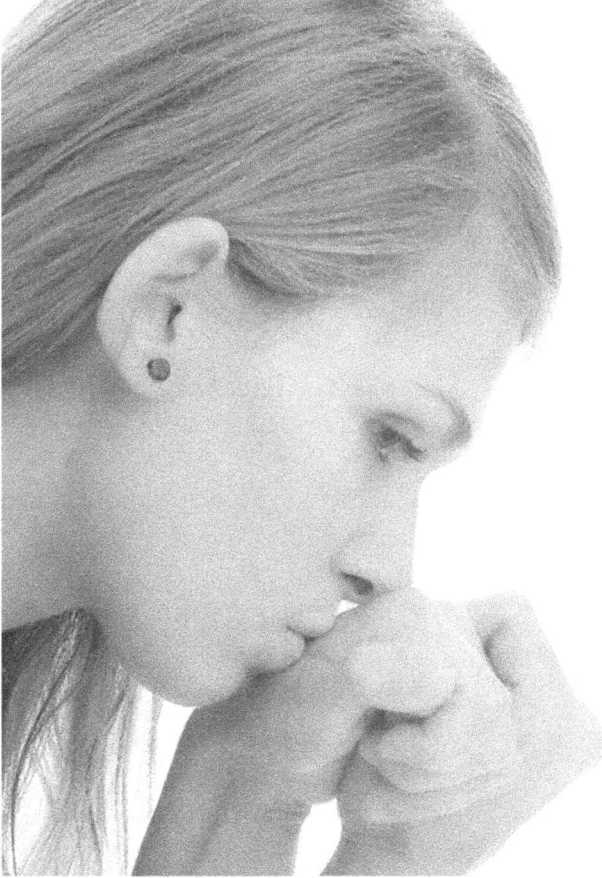

Dr. Val Jones was a medical student when it happened. Years later, as a fully accredited physician, she's still haunted by her inability to prevent the horror she saw unfolding before her eyes. In a post on her Better Health blog, she described how it began.

When I was a third-year medical student I was assigned to tag along with an ophthalmology resident serving his first year of residency as an intern in general surgery. We were to cover the ER consult service one night, and our first patient was a young Hispanic girl with abdominal pain. It was suspected that she may have had appendicitis. Part of the physical exam required that we rule out a gynecologic cause of the pain. And so a pelvic exam was planned for this young girl of about 12 or 13.

Remember what I said earlier about some hospital practices needing thoughtful revision? Few are as brutally intrusive as a pelvic exam. Would disaster have followed if that hospital had abandoned "staff are not male or female" for situations such as this and particularly for girls this young? This wasn't life or death. The formality of a rule-out pelvic exam could have waited until the next morning and the arrival of an experienced woman physician or nurse practitioner. Instead, we have what follows.

> She was frightened and clinging to her grandmother. She had never seen a gynecologist before and had explained through her grandmother that she was a virgin—making a gynecologic cause of her abdominal pain less likely. I offered her some reassurance with my broken Spanish and held her hand as we wheeled her on a stretcher to a private examining room. The resident whispered in my ear, "This is going to be fun."

That snide remark was the first warning Val got that something terrible was about to happen. Keep in mind the difficulties she faces. Medical students often idealize their chosen profession. Their first encounters with its mistakes and misbehavior can be difficult to accept. Val must absorb that what she is seeing is taking place in a hospital, and that it's being done by someone who should be her role model. That's not easy. I worked for about three months on Hem-Onc—that's about five hundred hours—before I realized that I needed to adopt a more questioning, assertive attitude. Patient care could go wrong, and when it did I had a responsibility to act. That's why we should treat Val's reticence with sympathy. At that point, she may have had only a few dozen hours in a hospital, not enough to develop a healthy skepticism, much less the far more difficult skills required to stop stupidity or worse. Worse soon happens.

> The resident was creepy at every stage of the exam. He was clearly relishing the process, slowly instructing the poor girl to position herself correctly on the table. He held her knees apart as she whimpered and cried. He pretended to have difficulty positioning the speculum, inserting and reinserting it an

unconscionable number of times. All-in-all it probably took ten minutes for him to get a cervical sample (this usually takes under 60 seconds). He performed the bi-manual portion of the exam in a bizarre, sexualized manner. I was furious and nauseated.

Clearly, this resident—let's call him Dr. Pervert—was a sociopath. He's devoid of a conscience. He feels no guilt and has no standards of right and wrong. He even gloated about what he had done later when he talked to the unfortunate Val. In his twisted mind, he thought his misbehavior would impress Val, a pretty young medical student. He could not have been more wrong.

The patient was finally returned to her grandmother and the resident took me aside to ask how I thought he did. The perverted expression on his face was not lost on me. I looked at him with daggers in my eyes, but I knew that if I confronted him head-on it could trigger an investigation and in the end I had no hard evidence to prove that he had done anything wrong. It would wind up being a "he said, she said" scenario. I mustered the courage to say, "I think you were slow."

For a fleeting moment he was taken aback by my insubordinate criticism and then he said the sentence that still haunts me today, "Well it was her first time."

Ponder for a moment the dreadful situation that Val found herself in. In an investigation, she would have pitted her word against his, with officialdom inclined to regard what she said as "insubordinate criticism." It's even possible that, if that little girl and her family became aware of the controversy, admitting Dr. Pervert was an actual pervert might been costly. Even if Val had spoken out, would she have accomplished anything? Not likely. Here's how she looks back on that experience.

Each time I think of this interaction I feel sick to my stomach. I wonder what more I could have done. I wonder if he is still out there violating his patients, and if anyone has ever confronted him. My only consolation, I suppose, is that he did not go on to become an Ob/Gyn. As an ophthalmologist one would hope that he had fewer opportunities for sexual abuse of patients.

I guess you could say that in my medical training, I witnessed a child rape. I don't think it gets much worse than that… and I don't know what to do with this horrific memory. I am forever changed.

It is my hope that these sorts of situations become true "never events" and that we create a protective environment where there are no career consequences for medical students thrust into the unfortunate position of whistle blower.....

Note that I never saw this resident again. Our paths did not cross after the incident, and it was only at the end of the exam that I fully recognized the evil of his intent.

She and I fully agree on the need for change in how medicine and nursing are practiced. Her hope "that we create a protective environment where there are no career consequences for medical students thrust into the unfortunate position of whistle blower," illustrates why I wrote this book.

Our perspectives differ though. In that blog posting, Dr. Jones relives an experience she had as a third-year medical student. In this book I relive my everyday experiences working on the nursing staff at a major children's hospital. We see the same issues from different angles.

Dr. Jones wrote about one big thing. I've written about a host of smaller ones. That's why I believe that protective environment should begin with everyday care by all staff and that policies and practices should be amended to prevent horrors like these from ever occurring. Prevention is always better than after-the-fact accusations that may or may not be handled well.

This book illustrates that. As a nursing assistant, I had more opportunity for mischief than most physicians. I spent hours every day with those post-op girls. Yes, I bent over backwards to make them comfortable. My reward was their trust. But to a great extent that protective environment began and ended with me, with only limited oversight from busy nurses.

Did the administration reward my efforts? Not in the slightest. Some in its lower ranks had left floor nursing because they had little sympathy for patients. All that mattered to them were task-completed numbers. I had to become a quiet rebel, doing what I thought best and relying on other staff to back me up.

My situation was not unique. For all too long, hospitals have failed to deal with embarrassment issues. The various cultural pathologies aren't hard to diagnosis. They begin with two rules, rigidly applied and of doubtful value, and result in a series of harmful behaviors. We'll take a look at them now.

First, there's the lie that staff are not male or female. That's why no structural impediment existed to prevent Dr. Pervert from performing an exam on this frightened young girl, even though she clearly did not want a man to do that. Take special note that everything that little girl feared and more happened. She was right, and the hospital was wrong—vilely and inexcusably wrong.

The horrors that little girl experienced are part of a continuum. When Maria asked her nurse for a bedpan and that nurse passed the task on to me, according to that widely accepted lie nothing of consequence happened. Yes, it's true that Maria took what happened well, but that same inability to distinguish male staff from female also explains the horrors that Dr. Jones described. Like it or not, the two are linked by a common and wrong-headed belief.

That needs to change. Hospitals should quit implicitly telling patients, "Whether our staff are male or female is irrelevant. You have no right to make demands of that sort." If a staff's sex matters to patients, then it should matter to hospitals. When that's not done, those like Dr. Pervert are licensed to do evil.

No, I'm not arguing for sexual apartheid, where staff only care for patients of their own sex. I know that wouldn't work, and that's not what I did. During my ten months on Teens, I handled as many embarrassing tasks for girls as I did for boys. But I did that knowing that my female patients saw me as different and took that into account. Staff women can do the same with male patients. Even a little effort will make a big difference.

Second, there's an assumption that medical necessity overrides all other considerations. Dr. Jones referred to that when she pointed out that the girl's abdominal pain required a pelvic exam. That's true, but that necessity didn't mean that the exam had to be done by this particular doctor at this specific time.

That needs to change. Alternatives are almost always possible and should always be considered as part of the process. Questions such as, "She is young and vulnerable. Can we get a woman to do this?," should be as much a part of formal decision making as, "We need to rule out a pelvic infection. When can we get an exam room?" Those considerations should be hardwired into policies and procedures, rather than merely tacked on as discretionary.

Third, hospitals use those rules to bully patients, making them less cooperative. We saw that with the events that so disturbed Dr. Jones. The young Hispanic girl and her grandmother were right to be suspicious of Dr. Pervert. Yet their objections were shoved aside, the girl separated from her grandmother, and that obscenity of a pelvic exam carried out. That bullying not only took time, it almost certainly created suspicions that brought more delays later. That girl will never forget what was done to her. Even years later, caregivers may wonder why she seems so frightened. That incident is why.

Being careful will have major benefits. To give an example, how much longer did it take me to be cautious for that first suture check on a new girl? Perhaps ten seconds more than rushing up (obviously male), muttering, "I need to check your incision" (medical necessity), and flipping up her gown up far more than she might like (other considerations). Yes, my approach took longer, but that was more than compensated for by having a more cooperative patient during her entire stay. Taking more time at the start saved time later.

That's why we should question whether those two rules and the bullying that results actually achieve the time-saving efficiencies that are their purpose. Suspicious, imposed-upon patients resist staff and delay treatment. Bully once, and you have to bully over and over again. That wastes time and costs money.

Fourth, focusing on bullying keeps staff from discovering better ways. How often had young girls been pressured into traumatic pelvic exams at the hospital that Dr. Jones describes? I shudder to think. Why didn't it consider alternatives? Because rules and bullying do work after a fashion. They do get patients to comply in the short term. But they also keep staff from discovering better ways that would result in happier and more cooperative patients. Hospitals and staff should take a serious look at practices that embarrass and see how they can be improved. That's what I found myself doing—and I was glad I did.

Keep in mind the issues I faced caring for those teen girls. Almost without exception, all were good patients, eager to cooperate and willing to give me, even as a guy, a chance. That's why I loved working with them. But all had an *embarrassment threshold*, beyond which they were uncomfortable. Even the first post-op girls, so casual with their gowns, hated linen changes. Others were even more cautious in differing ways. For some, wearing undies made bedpan calls acceptable. For others, kicking down their sheets to stay cool was their limit. Still others made me feel wonderfully masculine, as they peeked out at me sweetly from beneath sheets drawn up to their chins and requested a nurse for some mysterious purpose. Those differences, which at first confused me, proved easily handled, in part by giving them as many choices as possible.

Ah, but I faced another limit that came from giving choices—a *nurse's threshold*. I've mention it before. The embarrassing stuff was my responsibility. The nurse I was working with could handle only a small portion. That meant I needed to persuade perhaps eighty to ninety percent of those needs to come to me. Much of this book has been about how I accomplished that. Here I'll detail why my efforts worked and why similar efforts should work for you.

First, keep in mind a difference. I juggled a dozen patients and faced constant interruptions that left me little time to think. These girls had little to do and my visits were almost their only entertainment. That left them time to observe and decide if I could be trusted. In short, they were thinking patients. I never forgot that.

Second, embarrassment was *a factor* in their thinking, but not the only one. A miserably hot room mattered, as did a desire to show independence from a mother. They weighed all the factors, including my behavior, and reached a conclusion. Taking care with what I did brought more cooperation.

Third, necessity mattered to them. I knew why they hated linen changes. There was no necessity for me to do them, so I didn't. On the other hand, I did not hesitate with gown changes. I knew that even the most modest girls would recognize the importance of quick action. They cooperated even before my embarrassment-free technique brought those smiles.

Are you getting my point? These girls—and by extension your patients—were almost all reasonable and practical. My efforts to ease their concerns made them were more willing to move from cautious to cooperating. That's how I managed to stay inside their embarrassment threshold without crossing a nurse's threshold.

Ah, but there was a hitch. We've been talking about almost all my female patients while neglecting a large category of other patients along with some special cases.

Fifth, focusing on bullying prevents staff from responding correctly to those who need to be treated differently. I've told you about two groups where my efforts achieved little. I'll close with a plea to alleviate their plight.

You know about the misery of the first. All too many of our teen boys were withdrawn and unhappy. Their resistance to embarrassment was a symptom of a larger problem—their frustration with being treated as little boys. Our inability understand that wasn't surprising. We specialized in caring for children and thus failed to see that teen boys needed to be treated differently. That should change.

You've also met the other group. To understand it, remember that *most* of the girls I cared for, even the most modest, were strong and adaptable. They could see linen changes were stupid and hated them. Yet even though it meant more exposure, they easily accepted gown changes because those made sense and were done properly. Their dominant emotion was good sense. Treated well, they were happy and cooperative.

But there was another group of girls—fortunately far fewer in number—who did not adapt as easily. Their ruling emotions were fear and powerlessness. They had an intense concern for their modesty, but lacked the resolve to defend it. For some, their motivation was linked to culture or religion. For others, it result from sexual abuse. In every case, their embarrassment threshold was low and triggered an intense response.

The Min I cared for was one, and the young girl that Dr. Jones mentioned was another. Was there anything I could have done to ease Min's fears as I flipped her over? No, I was as careful as possible and her sheet never slipped, and yet that wasn't enough. Her fears went well beyond any assurance I might offer. Does it make sense to assume that, with but a little additional persuasion, the young girl Dr. Jones mentions could have come to accept any male examiner, much less one as creepy as Dr. Pervert? A thousand times no.

Those two girls did express their feelings. Min's fears were obvious, and Val's patient repeatedly protested. Unfortunately, these particular patients were unable to impose their wishes on a system already inclined to ignore protests. Their objections were shoved aside and their feelings violated. In today's context, the very patients that staff should be trying the hardest to protect are often the most easily violated. That's bad.

Staff can make a big difference with these patients, but they need support from their hospital. Min came just after I transferred to Teens. I like to think that if she'd come later, I would have had the confidence to ask her nurse to handle those flips. But staff should not have to summon their stubborn, rebellious streaks to do what's right. Support should be built into policies and practices, one example being that Very Sensitive Patient (VSP) status I mentioned earlier. A little effort will keep these uniquely sensitive patients from developing a life-long aversion to medical care that may cost them dearly.

Now I must go. I could add several additional chapters, mostly rambling observations about matters you can easily discover for yourself. But I've accomplished all I intended. My goal wasn't to dictate solutions to those whose experiences are greater than my own. Instead, I wanted to offer my own experiences to illustrate the variety of responses that patients have to embarrassment and suggest how staff can respond in practical ways. I want to encourage you to think about how to handle similar situations with confidence and skill.

In that, I hope I have been successful.

www.ingramcontent.com/pod-product-compliance
Lightning Source LLC
Chambersburg PA
CBHW022336280326
41934CB00006B/654